SEPSIS: SYMPTOMS, DIAGNOSIS AND TREATMENT

PUBLIC HEALTH IN THE 21ST CENTURY SERIES

The Anti-Inflammatory
Effects of Exercise
Pedro Tauler and Antoni Aguiló
2010. ISBN: 978-1-60876-886-8

Physical Activity
in Rehabilitation and Recovery
Holly Blake
(Editor)
2010. ISBN: 978-1-60876-400-6

Treadmill Exercise
and its Effects on Cardiovascular
Fitness, Depression and Muscle
Aerobic Function
Nuno Azóia and Pedra Dobreiro
(Editors)
2010. ISBN: 978-1-60876-857-8

COPD
Is/Is Not a Systemic Disease?
Claudio F. Donner
(Editor)
2010. ISBN: 978-1-60876-051-0

Research Methodologies
in Public Health
David A. Yeboah
2010. ISBN: 978-1-60876-810-3

Diarrhea: Causes, Types
and Treatments
Hannah M. Wilson
(Editor)
2010. ISBN: 978-1-61668-449-5

Diarrhea: Causes, Types
and Treatments
Hannah M. Wilson
(Editor)
2010. ISBN: 978-1-61668-874-5
(Online Book)

Scientific and Ethical Approaches
for Observational Exposure Studies
Alain E. Hughes
2010. ISBN: 978-1-60876-034-3

Strategic Implications
for Global Health
Maria Labonté
(Editor)
2010. ISBN: 978-1-60741-660-9

Influenza Pandemic - Preparedness
and Response To A Health Disaster
Emma S. Brouwer
(Editor)
2010. ISBN: 978-1-60692-953-7

PUBLIC HEALTH IN THE 21ST CENTURY SERIES

SEPSIS: SYMPTOMS, DIAGNOSIS AND TREATMENT

JOSEPH R. BROWN
EDITOR

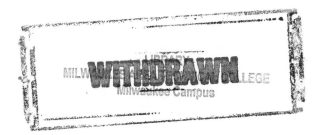

Nova Biomedical Books

New York

For permission to use material from this book please contact us:
Telephone 631-231-7269; Fax 631-231-8175
Web Site: http://www.novapublishers.com

NOTICE TO THE READER

The Publisher has taken reasonable care in the preparation of this book, but makes no expressed or implied warranty of any kind and assumes no responsibility for any errors or omissions. No liability is assumed for incidental or consequential damages in connection with or arising out of information contained in this book. The Publisher shall not be liable for any special, consequential, or exemplary damages resulting, in whole or in part, from the readers' use of, or reliance upon, this material. Any parts of this book based on government reports are so indicated and copyright is claimed for those parts to the extent applicable to compilations of such works.

Independent verification should be sought for any data, advice or recommendations contained in this book. In addition, no responsibility is assumed by the publisher for any injury and/or damage to persons or property arising from any methods, products, instructions, ideas or otherwise contained in this publication.

This publication is designed to provide accurate and authoritative information with regard to the subject matter covered herein. It is sold with the clear understanding that the Publisher is not engaged in rendering legal or any other professional services. If legal or any other expert assistance is required, the services of a competent person should be sought. FROM A DECLARATION OF PARTICIPANTS JOINTLY ADOPTED BY A COMMITTEE OF THE AMERICAN BAR ASSOCIATION AND A COMMITTEE OF PUBLISHERS.

LIBRARY OF CONGRESS CATALOGING-IN-PUBLICATION DATA

Available Upon Request

ISBN:978-1-60876-609-3

Published by Nova Science Publishers, Inc. ✦ New York

CONTENTS

PREFACE

Sepsis is a serious medical condition that is characterized by a whole-body inflammatory state (called a systemic inflammatory response syndrome or SIRS) and the presence of a known or suspected infection. The body may develop this inflammatory response to microbes in the blood, urine, lungs, skin, or other tissues. Sepsis is a leading cause of death in many intensive care units. In this book, the authors present and discuss current data on sepsis.

Chapter 1- Despite many years of extensive research and increasing knowledge about the pathophysiological pathways and processes involved in the septic cascade, the mortality rates from severe sepsis (documented infection-induced organ dysfunction or hypoperfusion abnormalities) and septic shock (hypotension not reversed with fluid resuscitation) in most centres remain unacceptably high. Ongoing research continues to provide new information on the management of sepsis. Importantly, there is increasing awareness that the syndrome is common, lethal and expensive and that it therefore warrants an organised, expert-provided approach to care. The treatment of severe sepsis and septic shock consists of prompt identification of the infection site, early and aggressive antimicrobial therapy, supportive protocols based on "early-goal directed therapy" and adjunctive therapies. In addition, a large number of immunomodulatory agents continue to be studied in both experimental and clinical settings in an attempt to unearth efficacious agents that reduce mortality. Eventhough initial preclinical results have been often promising, the majority of these trials failed to have any significant effect on septic patients when compared to other critically ill intensive care patients. Indeed cytokine orchestration, especially anti-tumour necrosis factor (TNF) and anti-interleukin-1 (IL-1) agents, has uniformly failed to lower the mortality rates of critically ill septic patients. In this review, we address promising research efforts that target blocking potential novel therapeutic agents including apoptosis, migratory inibitory factor (MIF), the complement split product C5a, ethyl pyruvate, bacterial lipoprotein tolerance and DAMPs (damage associated molecular patterns) including high-mobility group box 1 (HMGB1), heat shock proteins (HSP) and myeloid related proteins (Mrps). Notwithstanding previous disappointments with novel strategies, these inflammatory mediators show significant potential for the development of new experimental targeted therapies for the treatment of severe sepsis. We discuss in depth the reasons why successful in-vivo models and results do not automatically translate into in-vitro studies and deliberate why these newer agents should engender cautious optimism.

Chapter 2- Endotoxemia caused by Gram-negative bacteria can result in sepsis and organ dysfunction, which includes kidney injury and renal failure. The renal β_2-adrenoceptor (β_2-AR) system has an anti-inflammatory influence on the cytokine network during the course of immunologic responses. The previous reports indicated that the administration of β_2-AR agonists was found to attenuate the stimulation of renal TNF-α associated with lipopolysaccharide and Shiga toxin-2 of hemolytic uremic syndrome (HUS), which is considered to be a central mediator of the pathophysiologic changes. On the other hand, an altered expression and/or function of β_2-AR have been considered to be a pathogenetic factor in some disease states with inflammation; for example, heart failure and renal failure. These observations would suggest that blockade of functional β_2-AR activation might be associated with an increase risk for organ dysfunction following severe sepsis. In this chapter, we reviewed sepsis-induced renal injury and the genomic information to identify groups of patients with a high risk of developing sepsis-induced acute renal failure. In addition, we attempt to demonstrate a new insight into the immunological importance of β_2-AR activation in sepsis and an application of β_2-AR to septic renal failure and HUS. Furthermore, an *in vivo* β_2-AR gene therapy for the replacement of lost receptors as a consequence of sepsis was also described.

Chapter 3- Sepsis is a multifactorial disease for which the total number of cases is expected to reach one million in the United States by the year 2010. With the development of novel invasive surgical procedures, the number of sepsis cases has doubled in the past 20 years. Despite numerous randomized clinical trials involving tens of thousands of subjects, the effort to resolve the most challenging problem in intensive care remains elusive due to the complexity and rapid progression of the disease. Xigris®, the first FDA-approved drug for improving survival in patients with high-risk severe sepsis, failed to meet its high expectations due to its contraindications and its narrow label. There are also many examples of how recent research has led us astray. However, after a lengthy period of indecisive definitions of the disease, the healthcare industry is now addressing the major task of overcoming the unacceptable mortality caused by sepsis. This review provides an overview of medications that have not yet been approved for the treatment of patients with sepsis but have shown promise in clinical trials. These include drugs that target immunomodulation, the coagulation pathway, cell signaling, endotoxin, and specific mediators of sepsis. As the understanding of the disease has improved and the research into the development of therapeutic candidates has advanced, the expectations for a successful sepsis drug is now higher than ever. However, this will necessitate the development of an advanced diagnostic to specifically determine the condition of sepsis patients. The hope of providing relief to patients should encourage the healthcare industry to achieve these goals.

Chapter 4- Bacterial endotoxin (i.e., lipopolysaccharide [LPS]) elicits dramatic responses in the host, including elevated plasma lipid levels due to increased synthesis and secretion of triglyceride-rich lipoproteins by the liver and inhibition of lipoprotein lipase. This cytokine-induced hyperlipoproteinemia, clinically termed the "lipemia of sepsis," was customarily thought to involve the mobilization of lipid stores to fuel the host response to infection. However, because lipoproteins can also bind and neutralize LPS, we have long postulated that triglyceride-rich lipoproteins (very-low-density lipoproteins and chylomicrons) are also components of an innate, nonadaptive host immune response to infection. Once the lipid A portion of LPS inserts into the accepting lipoprotein, its ability to stimulate LPS-responsive cells is diminshed whereas its catabolism is increased. Furthermore, hepatic metabolism of lipoprotein-bound LPS results in an attenuated response of hepatocytes to proinflammatory cytokines, a process termed "cytokine tolerance." Several studies have shown that elevated plasma lipoprotein levels are protective against LPS-mediated toxicity in vertebrates. Recent studies have shown that apolipoprotein E, a component of plasma lipoproteins, is a key mediator of immunoregulation. Exogenous administration of apolipoprotein E increases mortality in a murine model of sepsis. Apolipoprotein E acts as a molecular chaperone for bacterial antigens, resulting in downstream Natural Killer T cell activation and cytokine secretion. Insight into the mechanism of lipoprotein-mediated immunomodulation has opened the door to potential novel treatment strategies of sepsis.

Chapter 5- In 2004, the Surviving Sepsis Campaign (SSC) was launched to improve the recognition, diagnosis, management, and treatment of sepsis. From that moment on a vast amount of articles concerning the early recognition and treatment of patients with sepsis and different tools to measure and improve the quality of care for patients with sepsis have been published. Although the SSC supplies tools to measure and improve the quality of care for patients with sepsis, no recommendations concerning the role of the nurses are given and effective implementation remains troublesome.

This chapter will mainly focus on the fact that early recognition and treatment of septic patients admitted to the ED can significantly improve after introduction of a predominantly nurse-driven sepsis registration protocol and education and feedback regarding its performance. An overview of the existing literature concerning general implementation techniques, focusing on different steps in the implementation process, is given. Apart from this overview, the effects of a predominantly nurse-driven prospective before-and-after intervention study at the emergency department are described. Compared to previous performed studies, this described new implementation technique was very successful. After the performance of the entire implementation program, four out of six recommendations and the compliance with the bundle of six recommendations improved significantly. It was demonstrated that four patient characteristics influenced the overall compliance rate to the sepsis protocol: patients' age, CRP result, ICU admission, and the final diagnosis.

In addition, following an educational intervention about sepsis, it was possible to improve residents' knowledge about sepsis definitions, and diagnosis and treatment of sepsis. Apart from the short-term effects, the improved test results were sustained after 4-6 months.

Chapter 6- Sepsis is a leading cause of death in many intensive care units. The pathophysiology is characterized by a dysregulation of the immune system in response to infection or secondary to a trauma. Initial hyperinflammation often results in septic shock.. Simultaneously, part of the immune system is deactivated leading to a temporary but often deadly immunosuppression. Recently, apoptosis of immunocompetent cells is being recognized as a key mechanism in the immunosuppression during sepsis. There is mounting evidence both in murine models and human patients, that apoptosis of lymphocytes, monocytes and dentritic cells is accelerated already in the early phases of sepsis. Inhibition of apoptosis in mouse models of sepsis by pan-caspase inhibition improves survival. Current studies suggest a role of both death receptors and the mitochondria in the initiation of apoptosis. Blocking the death receptor pathway with a fusion protein against Fas or by silencing the downstream caspase 8 results in a reduction of mortality after experimental induction of sepsis. On the other hand, protection of the mitochondrial integrity by over expression of the antiapoptotic protein bcl-2 improves survival as well. In humans, both an upregulation of Fas and a downregulation of bcl-2 are observed in lymphocytes of patients suffering from severe sepsis. In conclusion, the inhibition of accelerated apoptosis during sepsis is a promising target in the design of a novel and specific immunotherapy of sepsis.

Chapter 7- Sepsis is the term used to describe the body's systemic responses to infection. A consensus committee of American experts in 1992 defined sepsis as a systemic inflammatory response syndrome due to presumed or confirmed infection. Nonspecific symptoms such as tachycardia, leukocytosis and fever may be inflammatory in nature; when occurring in concert they constitute the 'systemic inflammatory response syndrome' (SIRS). SIRS occurring in a patient with proven or suspected infection is called 'sepsis' [1]. A review of the National Hospital Discharge Survey (U.S.A) data found that the incidence of sepsis increased by almost fourfold during the interval from 1979 to 2000, to 240 cases per 100,000 population per year [2].

Sepsis causes considerable morbidity, cost, health care utilization and mortality. Hospital mortality for sepsis patients ranges from 18% to 30%, depending on the series. While the mortality rate has decreased over the past 20 years, an increase in the number of sepsis cases has resulted in a tripling of the number of sepsis-related deaths [3]. There is a growing awareness of the need for an organized approach to caring for patients affected by sepsis. An early diagnosis of sepsis, prior to the onset of clinical decline, allows for prompt antibiotic administration and goal-directed resuscitation. The time to initiate therapy is thought to be crucial and the major determining factor for surviving sepsis [4,5], similar to the critical time-limit for early interventions in management of acute myocardial infarction and ischemic stroke.

In: Sepsis: Symptoms, Diagnosis and Treatment
Editor: Joseph R. Brown, pp. 1-27

ISBN: 978-1-60876-609-3
© 2010 Nova Science Publishers, Inc.

Chapter 1

SEPSIS: CURRENT TREATMENT MODALITIES AND FUTURE THERAPEUTIC TARGETS

Justin Kelly, Ronan A Cahill and H Paul Redmond

Dept of Academic Surgery, Cork University Hospital, Ireland.

ABSTRACT

Despite many years of extensive research and increasing knowledge about the pathophysiological pathways and processes involved in the septic cascade, the mortality rates from severe sepsis (documented infection-induced organ dysfunction or hypoperfusion abnormalities) and septic shock (hypotension not reversed with fluid resuscitation) in most centres remain unacceptably high. Ongoing research continues to provide new information on the management of sepsis. Importantly, there is increasing awareness that the syndrome is common, lethal and expensive and that it therefore warrants an organised, expert-provided approach to care. The treatment of severe sepsis and septic shock consists of prompt identification of the infection site, early and aggressive antimicrobial therapy, supportive protocols based on "early-goal directed therapy" and adjunctive therapies. In addition, a large number of immunomodulatory agents continue to be studied in both experimental and clinical settings in an attempt to unearth efficacious agents that reduce mortality. Eventhough initial preclinical results have been often promising, the majority of these trials failed to have any significant effect on septic patients when compared to other critically ill intensive care patients. Indeed cytokine orchestration, especially anti-tumour necrosis factor (TNF) and anti-interleukin-1 (IL-1) agents, has uniformly failed to lower the mortality rates of critically ill septic patients. In this review, we address promising research efforts that target blocking potential novel therapeutic agents including apoptosis, migratory inibitory factor (MIF), the complement split product C5a, ethyl pyruvate, bacterial lipoprotein tolerance and DAMPs (damage associated molecular patterns) including high-mobility group box 1 (HMGB1), heat shock proteins (HSP) and myeloid related proteins (Mrps). Notwithstanding previous disappointments with novel strategies, these inflammatory mediators show significant potential for the development of new experimental targeted therapies for the treatment of severe sepsis. We discuss in depth the reasons why successful in-vivo models and results do not automatically translate into in-vitro studies and deliberate why these newer agents should engender cautious optimism.

INTRODUCTION

Sepsis is present when there is clinical suspicion of infection combined with evidence of systemic inflammation. It is usually also defined by two or more of the following criteria: fever or hypothermia, leukocytosis or leukopenia, tachycardia, and tachypnea [1, 2]. Despite significant advances in our understanding of the molecular and genetic basis of sepsis and its associated immunologic response, sepsis remains a serious global problem as the primary cause of death in the noncoronary intensive care unit [3]. Despite many years of extensive research and increasing knowledge about the pathophysiological pathways and processes involved in the septic cascade, the mortality rates from severe sepsis (documented infection-induced organ dysfunction or hypoperfusion abnormalities) and septic shock (hypotension not reversed with fluid resuscitation) remain unacceptably high [4]. In the United States alone, it is estimated to be responsible for >100,000 deaths annually [5] with in-hospital mortality from sepsis rates fluctuating between 25% and 80% over the past few decades. Indeed, it causes as many deaths annually as those from acute myocardial infarction [6]. Although the crude mortality rate has decreased somewhat in recent years, patients with septic shock still have a higher excess risk of death than critically ill patients who are nonseptic [7-10]. Furthermore, it is also worth noting that the frequency of septic shock with multi-resistant strains is increasing.

Importantly, however, the concept that the syndrome is common, lethal and expensive and as such warrants an organised approach to care provided by experts is now more widely accepted [6]. A large multi-centre study, involving 192,000 patients, to determine the incidence, cost, and outcome of severe sepsis in the United States demonstrated an annual total cost of $16.7 billion nationally, with costs higher in infants, non-survivors, intensive care unit patients, surgical patients, and patients with more organ failure. Furthermore, the incidence was projected to increase by 1.5% per annum [6]. Previously, many physicians throughout the world were unhappy about the lack of a common definition for sepsis. One study highlighted the fact that 67% of physicians polled were concerned that a common definition is lacking and not more than 17% agreed on any one definition [11]. Thus, in an effort to improve communications related to sepsis and to allow early identification of patients with sepsis for possible enrollment into relevant clinical trials, an international sepsis definitions conference in 2001 was convened to summarize current definitions:

- Infection: a pathologic process caused by the invasion of normally sterile tissue, fluid, or body cavity by pathogenic or potentially pathogenic microorganisms
- Sepsis: infection, documented or suspected, and some of the signs and symptoms of an inflammatory response
- Severe sepsis: sepsis complicated by organ dysfunction
- Septic shock: severe sepsis plus acute circulatory failure characterized by persistent arterial hypotension despite adequate volume administration, unexplained by causes other than sepsis [12].

CURRENT TREATMENT MODALITIES FOR SEVERE SEPSIS

In 2003, a group of international critical care and infectious disease experts in the diagnosis and management of infection and sepsis met to develop guidelines that the bedside clinician could use to improve the outcome of severe sepsis and septic shock. This resulted in a comprehensive document created from the committee's deliberations being published [13]. Furthermore, the Surviving Sepsis Campaign, a joint effort of numerous professional organizations to expedite and standardize care of the patient with severe sepsis, was born from this endeavour [14]. The basic principle of this campaign is to create specific treatment "bundles" that individual hospitals could easily implement. The "Sepsis Resuscitation Bundle" outlines tasks that should begin immediately but must be done within 6 hours for patients with sepsis or septic shock and includes measuring serum lactate and obtaining blood cultures before broad spectrum antibiotic administration as well detailing guidelines for initial fluid management strategies and central venous pressure (CVP) targets in the setting of persistent hypotension. The "Sepsis Management Bundle" outlines those tasks that should be commenced immediately but must be done before 24 hours for patients with sepsis or septic shock. These include advice on steroids, recombinant activated protein C, glucose monitoring and mechanical ventilation [13-16]. The more salient features of some of these treatment modalities currently are discussed in the following sections.

EARLY-GOAL DIRECTED THERAPY

Early-goal directed therapy (EGDT) has been shown to improve survival by 15% in patients presenting to an emergency department with septic shock in a large randomised, controlled single centre study [17]. Up to 72 hours, those patients in the EGDT group had a significantly higher mean central venous oxygen saturation, lower lactate and base deficit concentrations, higher pH and lower overall APACHE II scores compared to those treated with standard therapy alone [18].

RESUSCITATION (FLUID THERAPY AND VASOPRESSORS)

Sepsis is associated with a profound intravascular fluid deficit due to a combination of vasodilatation, venous pooling and capillary leakage. Fluid therapy is aimed at restoration of intravascular volume status, haemodynamic stability and organ perfusion. The decision to use crystalloid or colloid as fluid resuscitation in sepsis remains a matter of intensive ongoing debate [15]. Despite data from multiple prominent meta-analyses of clinical studies comparing crystalloid with colloid resuscitation in the management of trauma and surgical patient populations, there is still no evidence based support for one fluid type over the other. This would appear to be generalisable to sepsis populations [17, 19, 20]. However, given that the volume of distribution is much greater for crystalloids than for colloids, it requires less colloid to achieve the same resuscitation end-points.

Initial resuscitation in patients with suspected severe sepsis or indeed evidence of sepsis-induced tissue hypoperfusion should begin once the condition is recognised. This is usually a clinical diagnosis but elevated arterial lactate levels reflect tissue hypoperfusion in those at risk who are normotensive. Also, lactate clearance levels early in the hospital course may indicate a resolution of global tissue hypoxia and is associated with decreased mortality rate. Patients with higher lactate clearance after 6 hrs of emergency department intervention have improved outcome compared with those with lower lactate clearance [21].

A simple four pronged targetted protocol will guide the physician in the initial steps in resuscitation with particular emphasis on

Central venous pressure: 8-12mm of Hg
Mean arterial pressure: >65mm of Hg
Urine output: >0.5ml/kg/hr
Central venous or mixed venous oxgenation: > 70% [14, 18].

Repeated fluid challenges that fail to manifest a clinical response are ineffective and should be avoided. There is less evidence to support the use of static preload parameters to predict fluid responsiveness in ICU patients so dynamic parameters (inspiratory decrease in right atrial pressure and respiratory changes in pulse pressure) should be used where available instead [22].

When an appropriate fluid challenge fails to restore adequate blood pressure and organ perfusion, therapy with vasopressor agents should be promptly commenced. Use of an arterial catheter gives a more accurate and reproducible measurement of arterial pressure. Either norepinephrine or dopamine is the first choice vasopressor agent for correcting hypotension in septic patients. Low-dose dopamine should not be used anymore for renal protection as part of the treatment of severe sepsis [14].

PHARMACOTHERAPY AND SOURCE CONTROL

It seems obvious that intravenous antibiotics should be commenced as soon as is possible. However, this should only happen when all of the appropriate cultures have been taken. Giving adequately broad empirical antibiotic regimes is also reasonable and full loading doses of each antibiotic should be given. Identifying the original source of infection is also of paramount importance as it may allow further control measures such as drainage of an abscess or local focus of infection. A large study comprising 2,731 adult patients with septic shock showed that administration of an antimicrobial effective for isolated or suspected pathogens within the first hour of documented hypotension was associated with a survival rate of 79.9%. Each hour of delay in antimicrobial administration over the ensuing 6 hrs was associated with an average decrease in survival of 7.6%. The relationship between hospital survival rates and the duration of time between the onset of hypotension and effective antimicrobial administration was similar in all major infection sites [23].

Despite thorough site culture specific sampling, findings may remain negative in up to 20% and blood culture findings are positive in only approximately 33% of patients [24]. However the finding of a positive blood or cerebrospinal fluid culture are considerably more significant than a positive urine or sputum culture result, as the latter are more likely to be contaminants. Inappropriate initial antimicrobial therapy is associated with adverse outcome in antibiotic-resistant gram-negative bacteraemia [25]. Delay of therapy has deleterious effects on clinical outcomes [26]. Conversely, de-escalating antibiotic therapy when culture findings are negative is a beneficial practice [27]. The microbiology of sepsis has also altered over time. Although in the past, gram-negative organisms were most commonly implicated, increasingly gram-positive organisms are isolated, such that roughly similar numbers of gram-positive and gram-negative organisms are now associated with sepsis [4].

INTENSIVE INSULIN/GLUCOSE THERAPY

Hyperglycaemia in patients in the ICU setting is associated with an adverse outcome. A large trial of postoperative surgical patients showed significant improvement in survival (mortality from 8% to 4.6%) when continuous insulin infusions were used to maintain glucose between 80-110 mg/dL. The protocol employed was relatively safe as there was a low incidence of iatrogenic hypoglycaemia and those in the tightly controlled group had fewer incidences of acute kidney injury, postoperative sepsis, ICU polyneuropathy and mechanical ventilation with the greatest differences seen in the sickest patients [28]. Another trial in a medical ICU conducted by the same group used 1200 patients who were predicted to remain in the ICU for at least 3 days. For those who remained for > 3 days (n=767), the results were comparable to the first study carried out. However, it was interesting to note that for those in ICU for < 3 days there was a significant increase in mortality rate in those treated with intensive insulin therapy (56 deaths) compared to 42 deaths in the conventional treated group. As it remains difficult to predict who will remain in the ICU longer than 3 days, some confusion persists about who should receive intensive insulin therapy although those dealing frequently with septic ICU patients on a daily basis will appreciate that they rarely stay < 3 days [29]. In some contrast to this group's experience, a large multi-centre German study (VISEP trial) was prematurely stopped as no benefit in mortality was seen in the intensive insulin group and frequent episodes of hypoglycaemia [30] were encountered.

STEROIDS

The applicability of steroid use in the ICU setting of sepsis has been debated intensely for many years. They have many potent anti-inflammatory properties including but not limited to; prevention of complement activation, inhibiting production of cytokines and interleukins, inhibiting the formation of inducible nitrous oxide synthase, enhancing the production of anti-inflammatory cytokine IL-10 from T-cells, preventing neutrophil aggregation and adherence induced by endotoxin and decreasing the release of adhesion molecules (ICAM-1 and VCAM-1). Steroids may also increase the number and sensitivity of α and β-adrenergic receptors and alter the release of proteolytic enzymes in the inflammatory process [31-36]. But the blanket use of high dose steroids in sepsis is not routinely justified as it has too many adverse outcomes [37, 38]. When examined as part of a trial of activated protein C, steroid-treated patients had a lower survival rate than those not treated regardless of treatment with activated protein C [39]. The use of low dose steroids now is strictly limited to those patients with septic shock and not in those with severe sepsis or other types of shock [14]. The

CORTICUS group found no difference in mortality or organ dysfunction in those treated with hydrocortisone or not [40].

As adrenal insufficiency plays a role in the pathophysiology of sepsis, the potential role of steroids in this particular subset of patients has been extensively studied. There is data available that supports the use of low dose steroid therapy in patients who have vasopressor-dependent type septic shock. A multi-centre RCT in France showed that septic patients who didn't respond to the corticotrophin test (having relative adrenal insufficiency) and treated with low dose steroid therapy for 7 days had improved survival rates without increasing adverse events. Non-responding patients with septic shock-associated early ARDS (acute respiratory distress syndrome) did better than those who were non-responders or who were in septic shock without ARDS [34, 41, 42]. A note of caution is advisable here as the practice of measuring patients' response to corticotrophin administration has been questioned. This is specifically because total serum cortisol depends on both the total free cortisol and that which is bound to albumin. Since albumin levels are commonly decreased in septic patients, they may therefore have a falsely low total serum cortisol level suggesting adrenal insufficiency in spite of normal free cortisol levels. There is also the significant issue in many hospitals that it takes numerous days before a result is available. Another problem is that some physicians remain sceptical whether a patient with relatively high cortisol levels would benefit at all from receiving additional glucocorticoid therapy just because they failed to raise an adequate response to an adrenocorticotrophin hormone (ACTH) test dose [43]. Thus, the use of the corticotrophin test is no longer advocated in septic patients [44].

RECOMBINANT HUMAN ACTIVATED PROTEIN C (RHAPC)

Drotrcogin alpha (DrotAA), a human recombinant form of the endogenous activated protein C that causes fibrinolysis and inhibits thrombin production, has been an exception among new therapeutic agents in that it has been shown to be successfull in reducing overall mortality from sepsis. In a large randomised, multi-centre, placebo-controlled trial involving 1690 people (PROWESS), rhAPC reduced the absolute mortality of patients with severe sepsis by 6% and reduced the relative risk of death by 19% [45]. A long-term follow up of these patients showed a persistent survival benefit 2-3 years after treatment [46]. Also, patients treated with rhAPC had a shorter time receiving vasopressors and requiring mechanical ventilation [47]. There is also evidence to support the swift introduction of rhAPC within the first day after severe sepsis has developed compared to the second day. This increased the survival rate and decreased the time requiring mechanical ventilation in the ICU [48]. It is suggested that rhAPC be given to patients at high risk of death (APACHE II > 25, sepsis-induced multiple organ failure, septic shock) and without absolute contraindications concerning bleeding. However, the ADDRESS study showed that it should not be given to patients with severe sepsis who have a low risk for death (APACHE II <25, single organ failure). These patients do not benefit from rhAPC but do have an increased incidence of serious bleeding [48, 49].

ANTIOXIDANTS

Antioxidants, especially high-dose intravenous selenium, are safe and recent evidence suggests their use to be beneficial in critically ill patients [50]. This was in a prospective randomized, placebo-controlled, multiple-center trial in Germany involving 249 patients with severe systemic inflammatory response syndrome, sepsis, and septic shock and an APACHE III score >70. Patients receiving selenium had an increased survival rate of 11.3% and no side-effects were attributed to selenium. Thus, treatment with high dose IV sodium selenite may reduce mortality rates in patients with severe sepsis or septic shock.

POTENTIAL NOVEL THERAPEUTIC AGENTS

A large number of immunomodulatory agents have been studied in both experimental and clinical settings in a number of randomised controlled trials in an attempt to unearth efficacious anti-inflammatory agents that may potentially reduce mortality. Eventhough initial preclinical results have been promising, the majority of these trials failed to have any significant effect on septic patients when compared to other critically ill intensive care patients. Indeed, in some cases, the trial agents led to increased mortality [51, 52].

For instance, cytokine orchestration has been widely studied, especially anti-tumour necrosis factor (TNF) and anti-interleukin-1 (IL-1) agents, however these agents have uniformly failed to lower the mortality rates of critically ill severely septic patients. Historically the most popular target fro sepsis treatment has been endotoxin or lipopolysaccharide (LPS) from gram-negative bacteria. Unfortuneately, numerous clinical trials using both the antibody-induced blockade of LPS during sepsis and monoclonal antibodies based on mouse or human tissue showed no substantial benefits [53, 54].

The most important factor to consider whilst determining the possible clinical benefits of successful in-vivo immunotherapeutic strategies is that these studies are usually conducted on purposefully bred cell line or young and healthy animals without overt disease [53]. In stark contrast to this, patients in the ICU setting are invariably morbidly unwell with multiple co-morbidities especially atherosclerosis and diabetes, thus exaccerbating and further complicating their systemic inflammation. In addition, in animal models, caecal puncture and ligation is classically used as the model to simulate an acute septic insult whereas the ICU patient, who may already have impaired organ dysfunction as a result of previously controlled chronic disease states, often suffers concomitant polymicrobial or multisite septic challenges. Labaoratory / animal based experiments also fail to account for human heterogeneity (including genetic polymorphisms) which may alter the clinical response to sepsis [53].

Here, below, we review the most recent promising research efforts regarding potential novel targets and pathways of potential therapeutic importance including apoptosis, migratory inibitory factor (MIF), the complement split product C5a, ethyl pyruvate, bacterial lipoprotein tolerance and DAMPs (damage associated molecular patterns) including high-mobility group box 1 (HMGB1), heat shock proteins (HSP) and myeloid related proteins (Mrps). In particular however, we also deliberate whether these inflammatory mediators seem likely to display any significant clinical promise for the development of new experimental targeted therapies for severe sepsis.

ANTI-APOPTOSIS AGENTS

Apoptosis, or programmed cell death, is the method by which tissue remodelling takes place during normal growth and development and is therefore the physiologic mechanism by which labile cell populations such as gastrointestinal epithelial cells, lymphocytes, dendritic cells, and neutrophils are regulated. It involves a series of biochemical events that lead to a variety of morphological changes including blebbing, changes to the cell membrane such as loss of membrane asymmetry and attachment, cell shrinkage, nuclear fragmentation, chromatin condensation, and chromosomal DNA fragmentation. Both the intrinsic (early activation of caspase-9) and extrinsic pathways (mediated through caspase-8) lead to activation of the "executioner" caspase-3 and a variety of proteases and endonucleases. Clinically, even though both apoptosis and necrosis are responsible for cell death during sepsis, it is widely recognised that the majority of cell death in these patients without severe reperfusion-ischaemia injury is due to apoptosis [54]. Patients who die of sepsis and multiple organ failure have lymphocyte apoptosis in the spleen, intestinal lamina propria and in lymphoid aggregates throughout the body [54].

Recently, numerous different studies have provided some evidence that using agents to inhibit apoptosis in lymphocytes thus blocking programmed cell death leads to improved survival rates in sepsis. Over-expression of the potent anti-apoptotic protein Bcl-2 in transgenic mice results in reduction of lymphocyte apoptosis and improved survival of animals [57-59], and inhibition of caspases prevents lymphocyte apoptosis and improves survival in a lethal model of sepsis [60]. Thus, the potential importance of apoptosis in the pathophysiology of sepsis is illustrated by results from animal models demonstrating that blocking lymphocyte apoptosis improves survival in sepsis. A variety of strategies to inhibit apoptosis may ultimately provide an effective therapy for sepsis.

MACROPHAGE INHIBITORY FACTOR (MIF)

Macrophage Inhibitory Factor (MIF) is a cytokine that was previously thought to have been produced solely by T-cells but was subsequently found to be produced by other cell types including pituitary cells, macrophages and monocytes [61]. Moreover, LPS, cytokines and glucocorticoids stimulate macrophages, T-cells and pituitary cells respectively to release MIF, causing an early peak level of MIF in sepsis. MIF then induces lymphocyte activation and antibody production as well as production of further cytokines such as IL-2 and IFN-γ. It also increases the production of other pro-inflammatory cytokines and chemokines by macrophages [62]. In addition, it can override the glucocorticoid-induced inhibition of macrophage and T-cell activation and can overcome glucocorticoid protection against lethal endotoxaemia [63].

High concentrations of MIF are present in the peritoneum of mice with bacterial peritonitis. Furthermore, wild-type mice treated with anti-MIF antibody are protected from lethal peritonitis induced by both caecal-ligation puncture (CLP) and E. coli, even when treatment is started up to 8 hours after CLP. Co-injection of recombinant MIF and E. coli markedly increases the lethality of peritonitis [64]. Also, mice deficient in MIF are resistant to the lethal effects of high dose endotoxin and have lower plasma levels of TNF-α compared with wild-type mice [65].

MIF has also been shwon to be an essential regulator of macrophage responses to LPS and Gram-negative bacteria. MIF upregulates the LPS-recognising Toll-like receptor-4 in an NF-κB-dependent manner, which leads to increased sensitivity of marophages towards LPS. When compared with wild-type cells, MIF-deficient macrophages are hyporesponsive to LPS and Gram-negative bacteria. Strategies targeting MIF have not been limited to gram-negative bacteria alone. Gram-positive exotoxins are extremely potent inducers of MIF secretion. Wild-type mice treated with anti-MIF antibody 2 hours before a lethal dose of gram-positive exotoxins improved survival rates by >45% [66]. These findings provide a molecular basis for the resistance of MIF-deficient mice to endotoxic shock and that MIF has potential as a target for therapeutic intervention in human sepsis [67].

Despite these promising experimental findings however there is some clinical ambivalence as to whether or not MIF levels are elevated specifically in septic/SIRS patients. One study showed a correlation between SIRS patients with high serum MIF levels and a poor outcome [68], whereas another study demonstrated no difference between MIF levels in septic and non-septic patients in an ICU setting when compared to a healthy cohort [69].

COMPLEMENT C5A

Activation of the complement cascade by either the classical, alternative or mannose-binding lectin pathways produces cleavage products C3a and C5a as well as the terminal membrane attack complex C5b-9 which ultimately cause cell lysis of target cells. The anaphylatoxin C5a is a potent chemoattractant that modulates the activity of numerous cell types including endothelium and bronchiolar epithelium [70]. It enhances the bactericidal and phagocytic activity of leucocytes [71] and causes the release of granular enzymes form phagocytic cells [72] and the induction of thymocyte apoptosis during sepsis [73, 74]. The production of C5a causes the downstream activation of NF-kappaB in a multitude of cell types [75-77]. Responses to C5a are initiated through the C5a receptor which is present on a variety of cell types and their expression is strongly induced during sepsis in the major organs including lung, liver, heart and kidney. Blockade of this receptor is highly protective from the lethal outcome of sepsis [78]. Animal models of this receptor activation have shown increased levels of intracellular adhesion molecule (ICAM) and vascular cell adhesion molecule (VCAM) on endothelial cells and induction of vasodilation and increased vascular permeability [79]. Recent data shows that IL-6 plays an important role in the increased expression of C5aR in lung, liver, kidney, and heart during the development of sepsis in mice and that subsequent interception of IL-6 leads to reduced expression of C5aR and improved survival [80].

Studies using a rat model show that injection of C5a closely mimics the systemic effects seen with LPS-induced sepsis. Furthermore, using specific blockers of C5a significantly decreases pathophysiological responses to LPS [81]. Blocking C5a prevents multi-organ failure [82] and protects rats from CLP induced sepsis and sepsis-related lethality [83]. In these studies, rats were either treated with C5a antibodies at the actual time CLP was performed to prevent progression to multi-organ failure or received neutralising antibodies directed against the receptor. When this treatment is delayed > 6 hours, as is seen in the latter case, then no survival benefit is seen. This suggests that a limited window of therapeutic opportunity exists immediately after the induction of sepsis. These animal studies also demonstrate the central role played by the complement activation system, by C5a in the pathogenic progression of sepsis in rats and that blocking C5a signalling could prove to be a particularly effective therapeutic strategy in sepsis [80].

In humans, blocking antibody specific for C5 has been shown to be a safe and effective inhibitor of pathological complement activation in patients undergoing ischemia and reperfusion of the heart (cardio-pulmonary bypass). One study demonstrated that C5 inhibition significantly attenuates postoperative myocardial injury, cognitive deficits, and blood loss [84]. Increased concentrations of the complement cascade products C3a, C4a, and C5a have been linked to poor outcome in sepsis [85, 86]. Thus, elevated plasma levels of complement activation products can be used to assist in early diagnosis of sepsis, to serve as markers for the severity of the disease, and to predict prognosis [87, 88].

ETHYL PYRUVATE

Ethyl pyruvate is a simple aliphatic ester derived from pyruvic acid and, in its role as an antioxidant, improves survival and reduces organ system damage in animal models of ischaemia / reperfusion injury, haemorrhagic and endotoxic shock. It also inhibits activation of pro-inflammatory transcription factors and down regulates secretion of a number of pro-inflammatory cytokines. It now would seem to certainly warrant evaluation as a therapeutic agent for sepsis in humans [89].

TOLL-LIKE RECEPTORS (TLRS)

Toll-like receptors (TLRs) are pattern recognition receptors which recognize distinct molecular patterns associated with microbial pathogens. Engagement of TLRs with their ligands leads to the production of various proinflammatory cytokines, chemokines, and effector molecules. TLR2 is mainly responsible for recognizing gram-positive cell-wall structures including Bacterial Lipoprotein (BLP). TLR4 is established as a signal-transducing receptor for LPS. TLR5 is the receptor for flagellin while TLR9 recognises CpG elements in bacterial DNA [90, 91].

An emerging wealth of evidence pointing toward a genetic predisposition in individual patients towards developing sepsis will have important ramifications in the clinical setting. Already studies have shown a clinical correlation between TLR4 and TLR2 polymorphisms in humans and the development of Gram-negative and Gram-positive sepsis, respectively [92, 93). Individuals with these naturally occurring polymorphisms represent an extremely high-risk population in terms of the development of postoperative sepsis, for whom, to date, no specific prophylactic measures exist. With future increased availability of genetic profiling and the use of genotype combinations it should become possible to preoperatively identify patients with TLR polymorphisms. This will allow the application of tailored prophylactic measures to prevent postoperative sepsis and morbidity [94-96].

BACTERIAL ANTIGEN TOLERANCE (BLP)

Antigen tolerance is defined as a reduced capacity of the host (in vivo) or of cultured monocytes/ macrophages (in vitro) to respond to antigen activation following a first exposure to this stimulus. The phenomenon of LPS tolerance has been investigated widely [97]. In vivo studies in our own laboratory have shown that induction of bacterial lipoprotein (BLP) tolerance, in addition to protection against a lethal BLP challenge, also protects against endotoxic shock through a cross-tolerance to LPS [97-99]. BLP tolerance results in a near-complete attenuation of pro-inflammatory cytokines including TNFα and IL-6, an increased polymorphonuclear population in the circulation and peritoneal cavity with over expression of dominant phagocytic receptors CR3 and FcγIII/IIR on both neutrophils as well as on peritoneal macrophages. We have also shown that BLP tolerance confers protection against lethal microbial sepsis induced by live bacteria or caecal ligation and puncture in wild-type and TLR4 -deficient mice via enhanced bacterial clearance [100]. Further identification and characterization of molecules in BLP and LPS signaling pathways responsible for BLP tolerance and its cross-tolerance to LPS are vital if we are to extend our understanding of molecular events involved during bacterial infection and associated septic shock.

DAMPs (DAMAGE ASSOCIATED MOLECULAR PATTERNS)

Pathogen-associated molecular patterns (PAMPs) interact with TLRs on innate immune cells to commence protective immune responses [101-103]. Damage-associated molecular patterns (DAMPs), which are intracellular components, such as high mobility group box 1 (HMGB1), heat shock protein 70 (HSP70), uric acid, the S100 proteins and cellular RNA released during cellular injury, also induce TLR-dependent inflammatory responses [104-107]. DAMPs also include any endogenous molecule, which undergoes a change of state (e.g. concentration or conformation) in association with tissue injury that can inform the immune system that damage has occurred [108]. These molecules are a unique group of intracellular proteins that when present in the extracellular matrix are recognised by the innate immune system as signals of tissue damage [109] and interact with cellular receptors expressed by various cells: by endothelial cells, resulting in inflammatory-cell recruitment, by epithelial cells, promoting the epithelial to mesenchymal transition that is important in wound healing and migratory behaviour and by immune cells, promoting pathogen recognition, or in the absence of pathogens, tissue repair. Many of these molecules promote the maturation of either tolerogenic or immunogenic myeloid DCs, depending on the nature of the other signals that are present.Whether the host is able to discriminate between DAMPs and PAMPs remains unclear. Although it is well established that the host can recognize "danger" induced by damaged tissue, it is unclear how an immune response that is triggered by a damaging insult is regulated [110].

Endogenous DAMPs activate a similar profile of cytokines and induce inflammatory responses similar to that induced by PAMPs. Significantly, some of these molecules, including HSP and HGMB-1 are not released during apoptosis, which is in keeping with the idea that programmed cell death is not a danger signal [111-114]. Whilst DAMPs represent an important aspect of defence against infection, they also represent a significant risk of inflammatory damage as evidenced by the fact that blocking certain DAMPs can be of benefit in treating inflammatory diseases [115]. The most relevant DAMPs to our topic are now discussed in greater detail.

(a) High-Mobility Group Box 1 (HMGB1)

HMGB1 was originally defined as a nuclear binding protein that is important for the regulation of gene transcription by stabilising nucleosome formation, however it was recently identified as a proinflammatory cytokine. It is secreted by activated macrophages [116, 117], mature dendritic cells and natural killer cells [118] in response to injury, infection or other inflammatory stimuli. Thus it has recently become known as a member of the DAMP family [119, 120]. HMGB1 is passively released from damaged or necrotic cells in infected or injured tissues [112, 121]. It binds to the cellular receptor for RAGE (advanced glycation end products), allowing activation of the transcription factor NFκB and mitogen-activated protein kinases (MAPK) [117]. Despite being host derived, HMGB1 can itself initiate TLR signalling, confirming itself as a danger molecule that can cause a second wave TLR-based signalling [106, 116, 118]. Activated macrophages secrete HMGB1 as a delayed and potent mediator of systemic inflammation [119, 120]. This release happens much later than the typical early release of classical pro-inflammatory mediators including TNF-α and IL-1. In a similar manner to other pro-inflammatory molecules, in moderate amounts, it will induce a benficial immune repsonse to confine infection, restrict tissue damage and promote wound healing. However in excessive amounts, it contributes to the uncontrolled inflammatory response that will lead to tissue injury and organ failure [109].

Currently three specific antagonistic modalities that target HMGB1 have been identified.

(1) Targeting HMGB1 directly with systemic anti-HMGB1-neutralising antibody leads to a significantly enhanced, long-term survival [120, 122, 123].
(2) Ethyl pyruvate, an experimental anti-inflammatory agent inhibits systemic HMGB1 release and rescues animals from the sequalae of systemic inflammation [124].
(3) Using the DNA-binding A box to inhibit endogenous HMGB1 reduces the lethality associated with already established sepsis [123].

Bacterial lipoprotein tolerance has also recently been shown to down-regulate HMGB1, representing a further novel means of reducing HMGB1 protein levels. This effect relates to a transcriptional down-regulation of HMGB1 gene expression, reduction in protein synthesis, and attenuation of HMGB1 secretion. It was also demonstrated how it is a critical factor involved in BLP-associated lethality, and that the targeting of HMGB1 affords almost complete protection against BLP-associated lethality [125].

Serum levels of HMGB1 peak at 8-12 hours after mice challenged with LPS or over 24-48 hours following CLP in mice, whereas peak levels of TNF-α occur at 2-4 hours [123, 126]. Furthermore, in humans, systemic cytokine release in sepsis has often returned to near normal states by the time an actual diagnosis has been reached [127]. Specific inhibition of these early cytokines that are released including TNF-α provides only a narrow window for possible clinical intervention. So broadening this window to include elements released later in the cascade such as HMGB1 may allow more succesful therapeutic strategies to be developed. Finally, it induces expression of VCAM-1, ICAM-1 and RAGE as well as secretion of TNF-α, IL-8, monocyte chemotactic protein-1, PAI-1 and tissue plaminogen activator. These findings link HMGB1 with the regulation of the complement cascade and adds further evidence to its potential use as a therapeutic strategy in patients with sepsis [128].

Giving systemic HMGB1 to animals does not cause shock in itself but it is still lethal mainly in part due to its disruption of the epithelial-cell barrier [123, 129, 130]. HMGB1 levels are markedly increased during severe sepsis in animals and humans, and passive immunisation with anti-HMGB1 prevents lethality from established sepsis in animals [123]. Unfortuneately, HMGB1-deficient mice die soon after birth as a result of lethal hypoglycaemia [131], so few significant animal studies have been carried out. However, unlike those who succumb to TNF-α-induced death, those that die from HMGB1-induced death have no evidence of haemorrhagic necrosis in the bowel, no marked responses in the kidney or lungs and no adrenal necrosis [123, 126, 132]. This almost complete absence of significant pathological findings is similar to the autopsy results of patients who died as a result of severe sepsis, as well as to the necropsy results of animals that died as a result of severe sepsis. This indicates that the effects of HMGB1 and TNF-α are plainly distinguishable and that these molecules are separate potential therapeutic targets in different clinical settings.

(b) Heat Shock Proteins

Heat shock proteins (HSPs) are a class of functionally related proteins whose expression is increased when cells are exposed to elevated temperatures or other stressing components [133]. They are secreted via a non-classical pathway and are also released by necrotic cells. HSPs function as intra-cellular chaperones for other proteins. Intracellularly they help to fold or unfold nascent or misfolded proteins, and assist in the establishment of proper protein conformation (shape) and prevention of unwanted protein aggregation. By helping to stabilize partially unfolded proteins, HSPs aid in transporting proteins across membranes within the cell [134, 135]. Extracellular and membrane bound heat-shock proteins, especially HSP70 are involved in binding antigens and presenting them to the immune system which allows the cross-presentation to the immune system of peptides associated with them [136].

HSPs are potent activators of the innate immune system. It has been shown that Hsp60, Hsp70 and HSP90 are capable of inducing the production of proinflammatory cytokines by the monocyte-macrophage system as well as the activation and maturation of antigen-presenting cells in a manner similar to the effects of LPS and bacterial lipoprotein, e.g. via CD14/TLR2 and CD14/TLR4 receptor complex-mediated signal transduction pathways [137]. HSPs seem to dampen the inflammatory process as illustrated by the inhibition of LPS-induced cytokine production in human monocytes overexpressing HSP70 [138]. They are present in the circulation of normal individuals [139], and their circulating levels are increased in a number of pathological conditions such as hypertension [140], atherosclerosis [141] and after open-heart surgery [142]. Specifically, HSP60 and HSP70 have been implicated in the pathogenesis of a number of autoimmune diseases and inflammatory conditions such as type 1 diabetes [143], Crohn's disease [144], atherosclerosis [145] and juvenile chronic arthritis [146]. Future emphasis of the interactions of HSPs with microbial molecules and the modulation of their inflammatory activities should open new horizons in our understanding of the complex mechanisms involved in sepsis.

(c) Myeloid_Related Proteins or S100 Proteins

S100 proteins (also known as myeloid-related proteins or calgranulins) represent a group of more than 20 calcium-binding proteins. The most prominent of these molecules are S100A8 (MRP8), S100A9 (MRP14) and S100A12. MRP8 and MRP14 form noncovalent homodimers and a heterodimer (MRP8/14) in a calcium-dependent manner [147, 148]. It is this combined complex of MRP8 and MRP14 that are the physiologically relevant forms of these proteins [149-152]. They are secreted by a nonclassical pathway [153] and represent the most abundant cytoplasmic proteins of neutrophils and monocytes [149, 150, 154]. MRP8 and MRP14 are secreted by phagocytes at sites of inflammation [155] and both molecules have pro-inflammatory effects [153, 156]. MRP8/14 is released by neutrophils, activated monocytes, and macrophages [150, 153, 157-160]. Both moelcules have been shown to regulate neutrophil, monocyte, or lymphocyte migration [161-163] and they are potently chemotactic for neutrophils and monocytes [164, 165]. Extracellularly, MRP8, MRP14 and the MRP8/14 complex all mediate regulatory and biological functions, including anti-proliferative, anti-tumoral, anti-microbial, and anti-nociceptive activities [166-171].

After release at local sites of inflammation [149, 155, 172-174], MRPs perform as DAMPs and can exert intra and extra-cellular effects. Faecal S100A12 has been reported to be an even more accurate faecal marker of inflammation than other previously used techniques when differentiating between inflammaotry bowel disease and functional bowel disorders [175]. There is a strong association between MRP8/14 complex and its potential use as a novel biomarker in a myriad of pertinent disorders including inflammatory bowel disease [176, 177], atherosclerosis [178], vasculitis [179, 180], SLE [181] and rheumatoid arthritis [173, 174, 182, 183].

Vogl et al demonstrated that Mrp8 and Mrp14 represent a molecular system involved in the pathogenesis of septic shock upstream of TNF-α induction [184]. They showed that mice lacking Mrp8/14 complexes are protected from endotoxin-induced lethal shock and Escherichia coli–induced abdominal sepsis. Mrp8/14 complexes amplify the endotoxin-triggered inflammatory responses of phagocytes. Mrp8 is the active component that induces intracellular translocation of myeloid differentiation primary response protein 88 and activation of interleukin-1 receptor–associated kinase-1 and nuclear factor-B, resulting in elevated expression of TNF-α. TNF-α induction is supposed to be a major effector of LPS toxicity [185]. However, blockade of TNF-α had a harmful rather than a beneficial effect in clinical trials of human sepsis, indicating that TNF-α independent mechanisms are major risk factors for sepsis, systemic inflammatory response syndrome and septic shock [186, 187]. This role may be mediated, at least in part, by MRPs in the manner indicated above.

Previously, it was unclear whether MRP8 exerts pro-inflammatory activities by itself. However studies have shown that human MRP8 possess pro-inflammatory activities toward neutrophils, and that recombinant MRP8, MRP14 and MRP8/14 stimulate human neutrophil chemotaxis, adhesion, and other pro-inflammatory activities, proving that they all exert activities toward neutrophils [164]. LPS-induced migration of mouse phagocytes has also been blocked by antibodies against MRP8 and MRP14 [165]. Thus, strategies that target these molecules might represent a new option for anti-inflammatory therapies. Taking into account the high abundance of MRP8 and MRP14 in inflammatory diseases, immune intervention that targets these proteins may be a successful strategy to block uncontrolled inflammatory processes. The inhibition of the release of these molecules may be another promising therapeutic approach.

CONCLUSION

Despite improvements in the overall understanding of the epidemiology and pathophysiology of sepsis, both morbidity and mortality remain unacceptably high. Numerous immunomodulatory agents have been studied in both experimental and clinical settings in an attempt to unearth efficacious anti-inflammatory agents that may potentially reduce mortality. In spite of promising initial preclinical results, the majority of these agents failed to have any significant effect. However, newer research efforts that target potential novel therapeutic agents including apoptosis, MIF, C5a, bacterial lipoprotein tolerance and some of the recently discovered DAMPs show significant potential for the development of new targeted therapies for the treatment of severe sepsis. Ongoing research continues to provide new information on the management of sepsis and possible specific interventions at a moleculo-pathological level therefore have given renewed optimism about further breakthroughs.

REFERENCES

[1]   American College of Chest Physicians/Society of Critical Care Medicine Consensus Conference: definitions for sepsis and organ failure and guidelines for the use of innovative therapies in sepsis. *Crit Care Med.* 1992 Jun, 20(6), 864-74.

[2]   Bone, RC. Sepsis, the sepsis syndrome, multi-organ failure: a plea for comparable definitions. *Ann Intern Med.*, 1991 Feb 15, 114(4), 332-3.

[3]   Parrillo, JE; Parker, MM; Natanson, C; Suffredini, AF; Danner, RL; Cunnion, RE; et al. Septic shock in humans. Advances in the understanding of pathogenesis, cardiovascular dysfunction, and therapy. *Ann Intern Med.*, 1990 Aug 1, 113(3), 227-42.

[4]   Friedman, G; Silva, E; Vincent, JL. Has the mortality of septic shock changed with time. *Crit Care Med.*, 1998 Dec, 26(12), 2078-86.

[5]   Mendez, C; Kramer, AA; Salhab, KF; Valdes, GA; Norman, JG; Tracey, KJ; et al. Tolerance to shock: an exploration of mechanism. *Ann Surg.*, 1999 Jun, 229(6), 843-9; discussion 9-50.

[6]   Angus, DC; Wax, RS. Epidemiology of sepsis: an update. *Crit Care Med.*, 2001 Jul, 29(7 Suppl), S109-16.

[7] Alberti, C; Brun-Buisson, C; Burchardi, H; Martin, C; Goodman, S; Artigas, A; et al. Epidemiology of sepsis and infection in ICU patients from an international multicentre cohort study. *Intensive Care Med.*, 2002 Feb, 28(2), 108-21.

[8] Annane, D; Aegerter, P; Jars-Guincestre, MC; Guidet, B. Current epidemiology of septic shock: the CUB-Rea Network. *Am J Respir Crit Care Med.*, 2003 Jul 15, 168(2), 165-72.

[9] Balk, RA. Severe sepsis and septic shock. Definitions, epidemiology, and clinical manifestations. *Crit Care Clin.*, 2000 Apr, 16(2), 179-92.

[10] Brun-Buisson, C; Meshaka, P; Pinton, P; Vallet, B. EPISEPSIS: a reappraisal of the epidemiology and outcome of severe sepsis in French intensive care units. *Intensive Care Med.*, 2004 Apr, 30(4), 580-8.

[11] Poeze, M; Ramsay, G; Gerlach, H; Rubulotta, F; Levy, M. An international sepsis survey: a study of doctors' knowledge and perception about sepsis. *Crit Care.*, 2004 Dec, 8(6), R409-13.

[12] Levy, MM; Fink, MP; Marshall, JC; Abraham, E; Angus, D; Cook, D; et al. 2001 SCCM/ESICM/ACCP/ATS/SIS International Sepsis Definitions Conference. *Crit Care Med.*, 2003 Apr, 31(4), 1250-6.

[13] Silva, E; Akamine, N; Salomao, R; Townsend, SR; Dellinger, RP; Levy, M. Surviving sepsis campaign: a project to change sepsis trajectory. *Endocr Metab Immune Disord Drug Targets.*, 2006 Jun, 6(2), 217-22.

[14] Dellinger, RP; Carlet, JM; Masur, H; Gerlach, H; Calandra, T; Cohen, J; et al. Surviving Sepsis Campaign guidelines for management of severe sepsis and septic shock. *Crit Care Med.*, 2004 Mar, 32(3), 858-73.

[15] Marx, G. Fluid therapy in sepsis with capillary leakage. *Eur J Anaesthesiol.*, 2003 Jun, 20(6), 429-42.

[16] Silva, E; Passos Rda, H; Ferri, MB; de Figueiredo, LF. Sepsis: from bench to bedside. *Clinics* (Sao Paulo). 2008 Feb, 63(1), 109-20.

[17] Schierhout, G; Roberts, I. Fluid resuscitation with colloid or crystalloid solutions in critically ill patients: a systematic review of randomised trials. *BMJ.*, 1998 Mar 28, 316(7136), 961-4.

[18] Rivers, E; Nguyen, B; Havstad, S; Ressler, J; Muzzin, A; Knoblich, B; et al. Early goal-directed therapy in the treatment of severe sepsis and septic shock. *N Engl J Med.*, 2001 Nov 8, 345(19), 1368-77.

[19] Choi, PT; Yip, G; Quinonez, LG; Cook, DJ. Crystalloids vs. colloids in fluid resuscitation: a systematic review. *Crit Care Med.*, 1999 Jan, 27(1), 200-10.

[20] Cook, D; Guyatt, G. Colloid use for fluid resuscitation: evidence and spin. *Ann Intern Med.*, 2001 Aug 7, 135(3), 205-8.

[21] Nguyen, HB; Rivers, EP; Knoblich, BP; Jacobsen, G; Muzzin, A; Ressler, JA; et al. Early lactate clearance is associated with improved outcome in severe sepsis and septic shock. *Crit Care Med.*, 2004 Aug, 32(8), 1637-42.

[22] Michard, F; Teboul, JL. Predicting fluid responsiveness in ICU patients: a critical analysis of the evidence. *Chest.*, 2002 Jun, 121(6), 2000-8.

[23] Kumar, A; Roberts, D; Wood, KE; Light, B; Parrillo, JE; Sharma, S; et al. Duration of hypotension before initiation of effective antimicrobial therapy is the critical determinant of survival in human septic shock. *Crit Care Med.*, 2006 Jun, 34(6), 1589-96.

[24] Bernard, GR; Wheeler, AP; Russell, JA; Schein, R; Summer, WR; Steinberg, KP; et al. The effects of ibuprofen on the physiology and survival of patients with sepsis. The Ibuprofen in Sepsis Study Group. *N Engl J Med.*, 1997 Mar 27, 336(13), 912-8.

[25] Kang, CI; Kim, SH; Park, WB; Lee, KD; Kim, HB; Kim, EC; et al. Bloodstream infections caused by antibiotic-resistant gram-negative bacilli: risk factors for mortality and impact of inappropriate initial antimicrobial therapy on outcome. *Antimicrob Agents Chemother.*, 2005 Feb, 49(2), 760-6.

[26] Lodise, TP; McKinnon, PS; Swiderski, L; Rybak, MJ. Outcomes analysis of delayed antibiotic treatment for hospital-acquired Staphylococcus aureus bacteremia. *Clin Infect Dis.*, 2003 Jun 1, 36(11), 1418-23.

[27] Micek, ST; Heuring, TJ; Hollands, JM; Shah, RA; Kollef, MH. Optimizing antibiotic treatment for ventilator-associated pneumonia. *Pharmacotherapy.*, 2006 Feb, 26(2), 204-13.

[28] van den Berghe, G; Wouters, P; Weekers, F; Verwaest, C; Bruyninckx, F; Schetz, M; et al. Intensive insulin therapy in the critically ill patients. *N Engl J Med.*, 2001 Nov 8, 345(19), 1359-67.

[29] Van den Berghe, G; Wilmer, A; Hermans, G; Meersseman, W; Wouters, PJ; Milants, I; et al. Intensive insulin therapy in the medical ICU. *N Engl J Med.*, 2006 Feb 2, 354(5), 449-61.

[30] Brunkhorst, FM; Engel, C; Bloos, F; Meier-Hellmann, A; Ragaller, M; Weiler, N; et al. Intensive insulin therapy and pentastarch resuscitation in severe sepsis. *N Engl J Med.*, 2008 Jan 10, 358(2), 125-39.

[31] Carlet, J. From mega to more reasonable doses of corticosteroids: a decade to recreate hope. *Crit Care Med.*, 1999 Apr, 27(4), 672-4.

[32] Kawamura, T; Inada, K; Nara, N; Wakusawa, R; Endo, S. Influence of methylprednisolone on cytokine balance during cardiac surgery. *Crit Care Med.*, 1999 Mar, 27(3), 545-8.

[33] Matot, I; Sprung, CL. Corticosteroids in septic shock: resurrection of the last rites? *Crit Care Med.*, 1998 Apr, 26(4), 627-30.

[34] Meduri, GU; Kanangat, S. Glucocorticoid treatment of sepsis and acute respiratory distress syndrome: time for a critical reappraisal. *Crit Care Med.*, 1998 Apr, 26(4), 630-3.

[35] Putterman, C. Corticosteroids in sepsis and septic shock: has the jury reached a verdict? *Isr J Med Sci.*, 1989 Jun, 25(6), 332-8.

[36] Schumer, W. Controversy in shock research. Pro: The role of steroids in septic shock. *Circ Shock.*, 1981, 8(6), 667-71.

[37] Bone, RC; Fisher, CJ, Jr., Clemmer, TP; Slotman, GJ; Metz, CA; Balk, RA. A controlled clinical trial of high-dose methylprednisolone in the treatment of severe sepsis and septic shock. *N Engl J Med.*, 1987 Sep 10, 317(11), 653-8.

[38] Zeni, F; Freeman, B; Natanson, C. Anti-inflammatory therapies to treat sepsis and septic shock: a reassessment. *Crit Care Med.*, 1997 Jul, 25(7), 1095-100.

[39] Levy, H; Laterre, PF; Bates, B; Qualy, RL. Steroid use in PROWESS severe sepsis patients treated with drotrecogin alfa (activated). *Crit Care.*, 2005 Oct 5, 9(5), R502-7.

[40] Sprung, CL; Annane, D; Keh, D; Moreno, R; Singer, M; Freivogel, K; et al. Hydrocortisone therapy for patients with septic shock. *N Engl J Med.*, 2008 Jan 10, 358(2), 111-24.

[41] Annane, D; Sebille, V; Bellissant, E. Effect of low doses of corticosteroids in septic shock patients with or without early acute respiratory distress syndrome. *Crit Care Med.*, 2006 Jan, 34(1), 22-30.

[42] Annane, D; Sebille, V; Charpentier, C; Bollaert, PE; Francois, B; Korach, JM; et al. Effect of treatment with low doses of hydrocortisone and fludrocortisone on mortality in patients with septic shock. *JAMA.*, 2002 Aug 21, 288(7), 862-71.

[43] Umpierrez, GE; Isaacs, SD; Bazargan, N; You, X; Thaler, LM; Kitabchi, AE. Hyperglycemia: an independent marker of in-hospital mortality in patients with undiagnosed diabetes. *J Clin Endocrinol Metab.*, 2002 Mar, 87(3), 978-82.

[44] Reinhart, K; Brunkhorst, F; Bone, H; Gerlach, H; Grundling, M; Kreymann, G; et al. [Diagnosis and therapy of sepsis. Guidelines of the German Sepsis Society Inc. and the German Interdisciplinary Society for Intensive and Emergency Medicine]. *Internist* (Berl). 2006 Apr, 47(4), 356, 8-60, 62-8, passim.

[45] Bernard, GR; Vincent, JL; Laterre, PF; LaRosa, SP; Dhainaut, JF; Lopez-Rodriguez, A; et al. Efficacy and safety of recombinant human activated protein C for severe sepsis. *N Engl J Med.*, 2001 Mar 8, 344(10), 699-709.

[46] Angus, DC; Laterre, PF; Helterbrand, J; Ely, EW; Ball, DE; Garg, R; et al. The effect of drotrecogin alfa (activated) on long-term survival after severe sepsis. *Crit Care Med.*, 2004 Nov, 32(11), 2199-206.

[47] Vincent, JL; Angus, DC; Artigas, A; Kalil, A; Basson, BR; Jamal, HH; et al. Effects of drotrecogin alfa (activated) on organ dysfunction in the PROWESS trial. *Crit Care Med.*, 2003 Mar, 31(3), 834-40.

[48] Vincent, JL; Bernard, GR; Beale, R; Doig, C; Putensen, C; Dhainaut, JF; et al. Drotrecogin alfa (activated) treatment in severe sepsis from the global open-label trial ENHANCE: further evidence for survival and safety and implications for early treatment. *Crit Care Med.*, 2005 Oct, 33(10), 2266-77.

[49] Abraham, E; Laterre, PF; Garg, R; Levy, H; Talwar, D; Trzaskoma, BL; et al. Drotrecogin alfa (activated) for adults with severe sepsis and a low risk of death. *N Engl J Med.*, 2005 Sep 29, 353(13), 1332-41.

[50] Angstwurm, MW; Engelmann, L; Zimmermann, T; Lehmann, C; Spes, CH; Abel, P; et al. Selenium in Intensive Care (SIC), results of a prospective randomized, placebo-controlled, multiple-center study in patients with severe systemic inflammatory response syndrome, sepsis, and septic shock. *Crit Care Med.*, 2007 Jan, 35(1), 118-26.

[51] Lopez, A; Lorente, JA; Steingrub, J; Bakker, J; McLuckie, A; Willatts, S; et al. Multiple-center, randomized, placebo-controlled, double-blind study of the nitric oxide synthase inhibitor 546C88: effect on survival in patients with septic shock. *Crit Care Med.*, 2004 Jan, 32(1), 21-30.

[52] Reinhart, K; Karzai, W. Anti-tumor necrosis factor therapy in sepsis: update on clinical trials and lessons learned. *Crit Care Med.*, 2001 Jul, 29(7 Suppl), S121-5.

[53] Esmon, CT. Why do animal models (sometimes) fail to mimic human sepsis? *Crit Care Med.*, 2004 May, 32(5 Suppl), S219-22.

[54] Hotchkiss, RS; Swanson, PE; Freeman, BD; Tinsley, KW; Cobb, JP; Matuschak, GM; et al. Apoptotic cell death in patients with sepsis, shock, and multiple organ dysfunction. *Crit Care Med.*, 1999 Jul, 27(7), 1230-51.

[55] Cohen, J. Adjunctive therapy in sepsis: a critical analysis of the clinical trial programme. *Br Med Bull.*, 1999, 55(1), 212-25.

[56] Ziegler, EJ; Fisher, CJ; Jr., Sprung CL, Straube RC, Sadoff JC, Foulke GE, et al. Treatment of gram-negative bacteremia and septic shock with HA-1A human monoclonal antibody against endotoxin. A randomized, double-blind, placebo-controlled trial. The HA-1A Sepsis Study Group. *N Engl J Med.*, 1991 Feb 14, 324(7), 429-36.

[57] Hotchkiss, RS; Swanson, PE; Knudson, CM; Chang, KC; Cobb, JP; Osborne, DF; et al. Overexpression of Bcl-2 in transgenic mice decreases apoptosis and improves survival in sepsis. *J Immunol.*, 1999 Apr 1, 162(7), 4148-56.

[58] Hotchkiss, RS; Tinsley, KW; Swanson, PE; Chang, KC; Cobb, JP; Buchman, TG; et al. Prevention of lymphocyte cell death in sepsis improves survival in mice. *Proc Natl Acad Sci U S A.*, 1999 Dec 7, 96(25), 14541-6.

[59] Iwata, A; Stevenson, VM; Minard, A; Tasch, M; Tupper, J; Lagasse, E; et al. Over-expression of Bcl-2 provides protection in septic mice by a trans effect. *J Immunol.*, 2003 Sep 15, 171(6), 3136-41.

[60] Hotchkiss, RS; Chang, KC; Swanson, PE; Tinsley, KW; Hui, JJ; Klender, P; et al. Caspase inhibitors improve survival in sepsis: a critical role of the lymphocyte. *Nat Immunol.*, 2000 Dec, 1(6), 496-501.

[61] Bernhagen, J; Calandra, T; Mitchell, RA; Martin, SB; Tracey, KJ; Voelter, W; et al. MIF is a pituitary-derived cytokine that potentiates lethal endotoxaemia. *Nature.*, 1993 Oct 21, 365(6448), 756-9.

[62] Calandra, T; Bernhagen, J; Mitchell, RA; Bucala, R. The macrophage is an important and previously unrecognized source of macrophage migration inhibitory factor. *J Exp Med.*, 1994 Jun 1, 179(6), 1895-902.

[63] Calandra, T; Bernhagen, J; Metz, CN; Spiegel, LA; Bacher, M; Donnelly, T; et al. MIF as a glucocorticoid-induced modulator of cytokine production. *Nature.*, 1995 Sep 7, 377(6544), 68-71.

[64] Calandra, T; Echtenacher, B; Roy, DL; Pugin, J; Metz, CN; Hultner, L; et al. Protection from septic shock by neutralization of macrophage migration inhibitory factor. *Nat Med.*, 2000 Feb, 6(2), 164-70.

[65] Bozza, M; Satoskar, AR; Lin, G; Lu, B; Humbles, AA; Gerard, C; et al. Targeted disruption of migration inhibitory factor gene reveals its critical role in sepsis. *J Exp Med.*, 1999 Jan 18, 189(2), 341-6.

[66] Calandra, T; Spiegel, LA; Metz, CN; Bucala, R. Macrophage migration inhibitory factor is a critical mediator of the activation of immune cells by exotoxins of Gram-positive bacteria. *Proc Natl Acad Sci U S A.*, 1998 Sep 15, 95(19), 11383-8.

[67] Roger, T; David, J; Glauser, MP; Calandra, T. MIF regulates innate immune responses through modulation of Toll-like receptor 4. *Nature.*, 2001 Dec 20-27, 414(6866), 920-4.

[68] Gando, S; Nishihira, J; Kobayashi, S; Morimoto, Y; Nanzaki, S; Kemmotsu, O. Macrophage migration inhibitory factor is a critical mediator of systemic inflammatory response syndrome. *Intensive Care Med.*, 2001 Jul, 27(7), 1187-93.

[69] Lehmann, LE; Novender, U; Schroeder, S; Pietsch, T; von Spiegel, T; Putensen, C; et al. Plasma levels of macrophage migration inhibitory factor are elevated in patients with severe sepsis. *Intensive Care Med.*, 2001 Aug, 27(8), 1412-5.

[70] Ward, PA. The dark side of C5a in sepsis. *Nat Rev Immunol.* 2004 Feb, 4(2), 133-42.

[71] Flierl, MA; Schreiber, H; Huber-Lang, MS. The role of complement, C5a and its receptors in sepsis and multiorgan dysfunction syndrome. *J Invest Surg.*, 2006 Jul-Aug, 19(4), 255-65.

[72] Goldstein, IM; Weissmann, G. Generation of C5-derived lysosomal enzyme-releasing activity (C5a) by lysates of leukocyte lysosomes. *J Immunol.*, 1974 Nov, 113(5), 1583-8.

[73] Guo, RF; Huber-Lang, M; Wang, X; Sarma, V; Padgaonkar, VA; Craig, RA; et al. Protective effects of anti-C5a in sepsis-induced thymocyte apoptosis. *J Clin Invest.*, 2000 Nov, 106(10), 1271-80.

[74] Riedemann, NC; Guo, RF; Laudes, IJ; Keller, K; Sarma, VJ; Padgaonkar, V; et al. C5a receptor and thymocyte apoptosis in sepsis. *FASEB J.*, 2002 Jun, 16(8), 887-8.

[75] Kastl, SP; Speidl, WS; Kaun, C; Rega, G; Assadian, A; Weiss, TW; et al. The complement component C5a induces the expression of plasminogen activator inhibitor-1 in human macrophages via NF-kappaB activation. *J Thromb Haemost.* 2006 Aug, 4(8), 1790-7.

[76] Pan, ZK. Anaphylatoxins C5a and C3a induce nuclear factor kappaB activation in human peripheral blood monocytes. *Biochim Biophys Acta.*, 1998 Nov 26, 1443(1-2), 90-8.

[77] Riedemann, NC; Guo, RF; Bernacki, KD; Reuben, JS; Laudes, IJ; Neff, TA; et al. Regulation by C5a of neutrophil activation during sepsis. *Immunity.*, 2003 Aug, 19(2), 193-202.

[78] Riedemann, NC; Guo, RF; Neff, TA; Laudes, IJ; Keller, KA; Sarma, VJ; et al. Increased C5a receptor expression in sepsis. *J Clin Invest.*, 2002 Jul, 110(1), 101-8.

[79] Schumacher, WA; Fantone, JC; Kunkel, SE; Webb, RC; Lucchesi, BR. The anaphylatoxins C3a and C5a are vasodilators in the canine coronary vasculature in vitro and in vivo. *Agents Actions.*, 1991 Nov, 34(3-4), 345-9.

[80] Riedemann, NC; Neff, TA; Guo, RF; Bernacki, KD; Laudes, IJ; Sarma, JV; et al. Protective effects of IL-6 blockade in sepsis are linked to reduced C5a receptor expression. *J Immunol.*, 2003 Jan 1, 170(1), 503-7.

[81] Smedegard, G; Cui, LX; Hugli, TE. Endotoxin-induced shock in the rat. A role for C5a. *Am J Pathol.*, 1989 Sep, 135(3), 489-97.

[82] Huber-Lang, MS; Sarma, JV; McGuire, SR; Lu, KT; Guo, RF; Padgaonkar, VA; et al. Protective effects of anti-C5a peptide antibodies in experimental sepsis. *FASEB J.*, 2001 Mar, 15(3), 568-70.

[83] Czermak, BJ; Sarma, V; Pierson, CL; Warner, RL; Huber-Lang, M; Bless, NM; et al. Protective effects of C5a blockade in sepsis. *Nat Med.*, 1999 Jul, 5(7), 788-92.

[84] Fitch, JC; Rollins, S; Matis, L; Alford, B; Aranki, S; Collard, CD; et al. Pharmacology and biological efficacy of a recombinant, humanized, single-chain antibody C5 complement inhibitor in patients undergoing coronary artery bypass graft surgery with cardiopulmonary bypass. *Circulation.*, 1999 Dec 21-28, 100(25), 2499-506.

[85] Hack, CE; Nuijens, JH; Felt-Bersma, RJ; Schreuder, WO; Eerenberg-Belmer, AJ; Paardekooper, J; et al. Elevated plasma levels of the anaphylatoxins C3a and C4a are associated with a fatal outcome in sepsis. *Am J Med.* 1989 Jan, 86(1), 20-6.

[86] Nakae, H; Endo, S; Inada, K; Takakuwa, T; Kasai, T; Yoshida, M. Serum complement levels and severity of sepsis. *Res Commun Chem Pathol Pharmacol.*, 1994 May, 84(2), 189-95.

[87]   Gardinali, M; Padalino, P; Vesconi, S; Calcagno, A; Ciappellano, S; Conciato, L; et al. Complement activation and polymorphonuclear neutrophil leukocyte elastase in sepsis. Correlation with severity of disease. *Arch Surg.*, 1992 Oct, 127(10), 1219-24.

[88]   Stove, S; Welte, T; Wagner, TO; Kola, A; Klos, A; Bautsch, W; et al. Circulating complement proteins in patients with sepsis or systemic inflammatory response syndrome. *Clin Diagn Lab Immunol.*, 1996 Mar, 3(2), 175-83.

[89]   Fink, MP. Ethyl pyruvate: a novel treatment for sepsis. *Novartis Found Symp.*, 2007, 280:147-56, discussion 56-64.

[90]   Opal, SM; Huber, CE. Bench-to-bedside review: Toll-like receptors and their role in septic shock. *Crit Care.*, 2002 Apr, 6(2), 125-36.

[91]   Vasselon, T; Detmers, PA. Toll receptors: a central element in innate immune responses. *Infect Immun.*, 2002 Mar, 70(3), 1033-41.

[92]   Lorenz, E; Mira, JP; Cornish, KL; Arbour, NC; Schwartz, DA. A novel polymorphism in the toll-like receptor 2 gene and its potential association with staphylococcal infection. *Infect Immun.*, 2000 Nov, 68(11), 6398-401.

[93]   Lorenz, E; Mira, JP; Frees, KL; Schwartz, DA. Relevance of mutations in the TLR4 receptor in patients with gram-negative septic shock. *Arch Intern Med.*, 2002 May 13, 162(9), 1028-32.

[94]   Arcaroli, J; Fessler, MB; Abraham, E. Genetic polymorphisms and sepsis. *Shock.*, 2005 Oct, 24(4), 300-12.

[95]   Stuber, F. Effects of genomic polymorphisms on the course of sepsis: is there a concept for gene therapy? *J Am Soc Nephrol.*, 2001 Feb, 12 Suppl 17:S60-4.

[96]   Villar, J; Maca-Meyer, N; Perez-Mendez, L; Flores, C. Bench-to-bedside review: understanding genetic predisposition to sepsis. *Crit Care.*, 2004 Jun, 8(3), 180-9.

[97]   Fan, H; Cook, JA. Molecular mechanisms of endotoxin tolerance. *J Endotoxin Res.* 2004, 10(2), 71-84.

[98]   Wang, JH; Doyle, M; Manning, BJ; Blankson, S; Wu, QD; Power, C; et al. Cutting edge: bacterial lipoprotein induces endotoxin-independent tolerance to septic shock. *J Immunol.*, 2003 Jan 1, 170(1), 14-8.

[99]   Wang, JH; Doyle, M; Manning, BJ; Di Wu, Q; Blankson, S; Redmond, HP. Induction of bacterial lipoprotein tolerance is associated with suppression of toll-like receptor 2 expression. *J Biol Chem.*, 2002 Sep 27, 277(39), 36068-75.

[100] O'Brien, GC; Wang, JH; Redmond, HP. Bacterial lipoprotein induces resistance to Gram-negative sepsis in TLR4-deficient mice via enhanced bacterial clearance. *J Immunol.*, 2005 Jan 15, 174(2), 1020-6.

[101] Janeway CA, Jr. Approaching the asymptote? Evolution and revolution in immunology. *Cold Spring Harb Symp Quant Biol.*, 1989, 54 Pt 1:1-13.

[102] Liu, Y; Janeway, CA, Jr. Microbial induction of co-stimulatory activity for CD4 T-cell growth. *Int Immunol.*, 1991 Apr, 3(4), 323-32.

[103] Medzhitov, R; Preston-Hurlburt, P; Janeway, CA; Jr. A human homologue of the Drosophila Toll protein signals activation of adaptive immunity. *Nature.*, 1997 Jul 24, 388(6640), 394-7.

[104] Cavassani, KA; Ishii, M; Wen, H; Schaller, MA; Lincoln, PM; Lukacs, NW; et al. TLR3 is an endogenous sensor of tissue necrosis during acute inflammatory events. *J Exp Med.*, 2008 Oct 27, 205(11), 2609-21.

[105] Millar, DG; Garza, KM; Odermatt, B; Elford, AR; Ono, N; Li, Z; et al. Hsp70 promotes antigen-presenting cell function and converts T-cell tolerance to autoimmunity in vivo. *Nat Med.*, 2003 Dec, 9(12), 1469-76.

[106] Park, JS; Svetkauskaite, D; He, Q; Kim, JY; Strassheim, D; Ishizaka, A; et al. Involvement of toll-like receptors 2 and 4 in cellular activation by high mobility group box 1 protein. *J Biol Chem.*, 2004 Feb 27, 279(9), 7370-7.

[107] Tian, J; Avalos, AM; Mao, SY; Chen, B; Senthil, K; Wu, H; et al. Toll-like receptor 9-dependent activation by DNA-containing immune complexes is mediated by HMGB1 and RAGE. *Nat Immunol.*, 2007 May, 8(5), 487-96.

[108] Wakefield, D; Gray, P; Chang, J; Di Girolamo, N; McCluskey, P. The role of PAMP's and DAMP's in the pathogenesis of acute and recurrent anterior uveitis. *Br J Ophthalmol.*, 2009 Mar 4.

[109] Lotze, MT; Tracey, KJ. High-mobility group box 1 protein (HMGB1), nuclear weapon in the immune arsenal. *Nat Rev Immunol.*, 2005 Apr, 5(4), 331-42.

[110] Papadimitraki, ED; Bertsias, GK; Boumpas, DT. Toll like receptors and autoimmunity: a critical appraisal. *J Autoimmun.*, 2007 Dec, 29(4), 310-8.

[111] Basu, S; Binder, RJ; Suto, R; Anderson, KM; Srivastava, PK. Necrotic but not apoptotic cell death releases heat shock proteins, which deliver a partial maturation signal to dendritic cells and activate the NF-kappa B pathway. *Int Immunol.*, 2000 Nov, 12(11), 1539-46.

[112] Rovere-Querini, P; Capobianco, A; Scaffidi, P; Valentinis, B; Catalanotti, F; Giazzon, M; et al. HMGB1 is an endogenous immune adjuvant released by necrotic cells. *EMBO Rep.*, 2004 Aug, 5(8), 825-30.

[113] Scaffidi, P; Misteli, T; Bianchi, ME. Release of chromatin protein HMGB1 by necrotic cells triggers inflammation. *Nature.*, 2002 Jul 11, 418(6894), 191-5.

[114] Vabulas, RM; Wagner, H; Schild, H. Heat shock proteins as ligands of toll-like receptors. *Curr Top Microbiol Immunol.*, 2002, 270:169-84.

[115] Mantell, LL; Parrish, WR; Ulloa, L. Hmgb-1 as a therapeutic target for infectious and inflammatory disorders. *Shock.*, 2006 Jan, 25(1), 4-11.

[116] Qin, S; Wang, H; Yuan, R; Li, H; Ochani, M; Ochani, K; et al. Role of HMGB1 in apoptosis-mediated sepsis lethality. *J Exp Med.*, 2006 Jul 10, 203(7), 1637-42.

[117] Wang, H; Yang, H; Czura, CJ; Sama, AE; Tracey, KJ. HMGB1 as a late mediator of lethal systemic inflammation. *Am J Respir Crit Care Med.*, 2001 Nov 15, 164(10 Pt 1), 1768-73.

[118] Yu, M; Wang, H; Ding, A; Golenbock, DT; Latz, E; Czura, CJ; et al. HMGB1 signals through toll-like receptor (TLR) 4 and TLR2. *Shock.*, 2006 Aug, 26(2), 174-9.

[119] Bonaldi, T; Talamo, F; Scaffidi, P; Ferrera, D; Porto, A; Bachi, A; et al. Monocytic cells hyperacetylate chromatin protein HMGB1 to redirect it towards secretion. *EMBO J.*, 2003 Oct 15, 22(20), 5551-60.

[120] Wang, H; Bloom, O; Zhang, M; Vishnubhakat, JM; Ombrellino, M; Che, J; et al. HMG-1 as a late mediator of endotoxin lethality in mice. *Science.*, 1999 Jul 9, 285(5425), 248-51.

[121] Watanabe, T; Kubota, S; Nagaya, M; Ozaki, S; Nagafuchi, H; Akashi, K; et al. The role of HMGB-1 on the development of necrosis during hepatic ischemia and hepatic ischemia/reperfusion injury in mice. *J Surg Res.*, 2005 Mar, 124(1), 59-66.

[122] Abraham, E; Arcaroli, J; Carmody, A; Wang, H; Tracey, KJ. HMG-1 as a mediator of acute lung inflammation. *J Immunol.*, 2000 Sep 15, 165(6), 2950-4.

[123] Yang, H; Ochani, M; Li, J; Qiang, X; Tanovic, M; Harris, HE; et al. Reversing established sepsis with antagonists of endogenous high-mobility group box 1. *Proc Natl Acad Sci U S A.*, 2004 Jan 6, 101(1), 296-301.

[124] Ulloa, L; Ochani, M; Yang, H; Tanovic, M; Halperin, D; Yang, R; et al. Ethyl pyruvate prevents lethality in mice with established lethal sepsis and systemic inflammation. *Proc Natl Acad Sci U S A.*, 2002 Sep 17, 99(19), 12351-6.

[125] Coffey, JC; Wang, JH; Kelly, R; Romics, L; Jr., O'Callaghan, A; Fiuza, C; et al. Tolerization with BLP down-regulates HMGB1 a critical mediator of sepsis-related lethality. *J Leukoc Biol.*, 2007 Oct, 82(4), 906-14.

[126] Wang, H; Yang, H; Tracey, KJ. Extracellular role of HMGB1 in inflammation and sepsis. *J Intern Med.*, 2004 Mar, 255(3), 320-31.

[127] Ulloa, L; Tracey, KJ. The "cytokine profile": a code for sepsis. *Trends Mol Med.*, 2005 Feb, 11(2), 56-63.

[128] Fiuza, C; Bustin, M; Talwar, S; Tropea, M; Gerstenberger, E; Shelhamer, JH; et al. Inflammation-promoting activity of HMGB1 on human microvascular endothelial cells. *Blood.*, 2003 Apr 1, 101(7), 2652-60.

[129] Sappington, PL; Fink, ME; Yang, R; Delude, RL; Fink, MP. Ethyl pyruvate provides durable protection against inflammation-induced intestinal epithelial barrier dysfunction. *Shock.*, 2003 Dec, 20(6), 521-8.

[130] Sappington, PL; Yang, R; Yang, H; Tracey, KJ; Delude, RL; Fink, MP. HMGB1 B box increases the permeability of Caco-2 enterocytic monolayers and impairs intestinal barrier function in mice. *Gastroenterology.*, 2002 Sep, 123(3), 790-802.

[131] Calogero, S; Grassi, F; Aguzzi, A; Voigtlander, T; Ferrier, P; Ferrari, S; et al. The lack of chromosomal protein Hmg1 does not disrupt cell growth but causes lethal hypoglycaemia in newborn mice. *Nat Genet.*, 1999 Jul, 22(3), 276-80.

[132] Czura, CJ; Yang, H; Amella, CA; Tracey, KJ. HMGB1 in the immunology of sepsis (not septic shock) and arthritis. *Adv Immunol.*, 2004, 84:181-200.

[133] De Maio, A. Heat shock proteins: facts, thoughts, and dreams. *Shock.* 1999 Jan, 11(1), 1-12.

[134] Borges, JC; Ramos, CH. Protein folding assisted by chaperones. *Protein Pept Lett.*, 2005 Apr, 12(3), 257-61.

[135] Walter, S; Buchner, J. Molecular chaperones--cellular machines for protein folding. *Angew Chem Int Ed Engl.*, 2002 Apr 2, 41(7), 1098-113.

[136] Nishikawa, M; Takemoto, S; Takakura, Y. Heat shock protein derivatives for delivery of antigens to antigen presenting cells. *Int J Pharm.*, 2008 Apr 16, 354(1-2), 23-7.

[137] Tsan, MF; Gao, B. Cytokine function of heat shock proteins. *Am J Physiol Cell Physiol.*, 2004 Apr, 286(4), C739-44.

[138] Ding, XZ; Fernandez-Prada, CM; Bhattacharjee, AK; Hoover, DL. Over-Expression of Hsp-70 Inhibits Bacterial Lipopolysaccharide-Induced Production of Cytokines in Human Monocyte-Derived Macrophages. *Cytokine.*, 2001, 16(6), 210-9.

[139] Pockley, AG; Bulmer, J; Hanks, BM; Wright, BH. Identification of human heat shock protein 60 (Hsp60) and anti-Hsp60 antibodies in the peripheral circulation of normal individuals. *Cell Stress Chaperones.*, 1999 Mar, 4(1), 29-35.

[140] Pockley, AG; Wu, R; Lemne, C; Kiessling, R; de Faire, U; Frostegard, J. Circulating heat shock protein 60 is associated with early cardiovascular disease. *Hypertension.*, 2000 Aug, 36(2), 303-7.

[141] Xu, Q. Role of heat shock proteins in atherosclerosis. *Arterioscler Thromb Vasc Biol.*, 2002 Oct 1, 22(10), 1547-59.

[142] Dybdahl, B; Wahba, A; Lien, E; Flo, TH; Waage, A; Qureshi, N; et al. Inflammatory response after open heart surgery: release of heat-shock protein 70 and signaling through toll-like receptor-4. *Circulation.*, 2002 Feb 12, 105(6), 685-90.

[143] Abulafia-Lapid, R; Elias, D; Raz, I; Keren-Zur, Y; Atlan, H; Cohen, IR. T cell proliferative responses of type 1 diabetes patients and healthy individuals to human hsp60 and its peptides. *J Autoimmun.*, 1999 Mar, 12(2), 121-9.

[144] Szewczuk, MR; Depew, WT. Evidence for T lymphocyte reactivity to the 65 kilodalton heat shock protein of mycobacterium in active Crohn's disease. *Clin Invest Med.*, 1992 Dec, 15(6), 494-505.

[145] Pockley, AG. Heat shock proteins, inflammation, and cardiovascular disease. *Circulation.* 2002 Feb 26, 105(8), 1012-7.

[146] Pope, RM; Lovis, RM; Gupta, RS. Activation of synovial fluid T lymphocytes by 60-kd heat-shock proteins in patients with inflammatory synovitis. *Arthritis Rheum.*, 1992 Jan, 35(1), 43-8.

[147] Barthe, C; Figarella, C; Carrere, J; Guy-Crotte, O. Identification of 'cystic fibrosis protein' as a complex of two calcium-binding proteins present in human cells of myeloid origin. *Biochim Biophys Acta.*, 1991 Feb 22, 1096(2), 175-7.

[148] Teigelkamp, S; Bhardwaj, RS; Roth, J; Meinardus-Hager, G; Karas, M; Sorg, C. Calcium-dependent complex assembly of the myeloic differentiation proteins MRP-8 and MRP-14. *J Biol Chem.*, 1991 Jul 15, 266(20), 13462-7.

[149] Foell, D; Roth, J. Proinflammatory S100 proteins in arthritis and autoimmune disease. *Arthritis Rheum.*, 2004 Dec, 50(12), 3762-71.

[150] Roth, J; Burwinkel, F; van den Bos, C; Goebeler, M; Vollmer, E; Sorg, C. MRP8 and MRP14, S-100-like proteins associated with myeloid differentiation, are translocated to plasma membrane and intermediate filaments in a calcium-dependent manner. *Blood.* 1993 Sep 15, 82(6), 1875-83.

[151] Vogl, T; Ludwig, S; Goebeler, M; Strey, A; Thorey, IS; Reichelt, R; et al. MRP8 and MRP14 control microtubule reorganization during transendothelial migration of phagocytes. *Blood.*, 2004 Dec 15, 104(13), 4260-8.

[152] Vogl, T; Roth, J; Sorg, C; Hillenkamp, F; Strupat, K. Calcium-induced noncovalently linked tetramers of MRP8 and MRP14 detected by ultraviolet matrix-assisted laser desorption/ionization mass spectrometry. *J Am Soc Mass Spectrom.*, 1999 Nov, 10(11), 1124-30.

[153] Rammes, A; Roth, J; Goebeler, M; Klempt, M; Hartmann, M; Sorg, C. Myeloid-related protein (MRP) 8 and MRP14, calcium-binding proteins of the S100 family, are secreted by activated monocytes via a novel, tubulin-dependent pathway. *J Biol Chem.*, 1997 Apr 4, 272(14), 9496-502.

[154] Roth, J; Vogl, T; Sorg, C; Sunderkotter, C. Phagocyte-specific S100 proteins: a novel group of proinflammatory molecules. *Trends Immunol.*, 2003 Apr, 24(4), 155-8.

[155] Foell, D; Wittkowski, H; Vogl, T; Roth, J. S100 proteins expressed in phagocytes: a novel group of damage-associated molecular pattern molecules. *J Leukoc Biol.*, 2007 Jan, 81(1), 28-37.

[156] Frosch, M; Strey, A; Vogl, T; Wulffraat, NM; Kuis, W; Sunderkotter, C; et al. Myeloid-related proteins 8 and 14 are specifically secreted during interaction of phagocytes and activated endothelium and are useful markers for monitoring disease activity in pauciarticular-onset juvenile rheumatoid arthritis. *Arthritis Rheum.*, 2000 Mar, 43(3), 628-37.

[157] Hetland, G; Talgo, GJ; Fagerhol, MK. Chemotaxins C5a and fMLP induce release of calprotectin (leucocyte L1 protein) from polymorphonuclear cells in vitro. *Mol Pathol.*, 1998 Jun, 51(3), 143-8.

[158] Lugering, N; Kucharzik, T; Lugering, A; Winde, G; Sorg, C; Domschke, W; et al. Importance of combined treatment with IL-10 and IL-4, but not IL-13, for inhibition of monocyte release of the Ca(2+)-binding protein MRP8/14. *Immunology.*, 1997 May, 91(1), 130-4.

[159] Pechkovsky, DV; Zalutskaya, OM; Ivanov, GI; Misuno, NI. Calprotectin (MRP8/14 protein complex) release during mycobacterial infection in vitro and in vivo. *FEMS Immunol Med Microbiol.*, 2000 Sep, 29(1), 27-33.

[160] Voganatsi, A; Panyutich, A; Miyasaki, KT; Murthy, RK. Mechanism of extracellular release of human neutrophil calprotectin complex. *J Leukoc Biol.*, 2001 Jul, 70(1), 130-4.

[161] Hofmann, MA; Drury, S; Fu, C; Qu, W; Taguchi, A; Lu, Y; et al. RAGE mediates a novel proinflammatory axis: a central cell surface receptor for S100/calgranulin polypeptides. *Cell.* 1999 Jun 25, 97(7), 889-901.

[162] Lackmann, M; Cornish, CJ; Simpson, RJ; Moritz, RL; Geczy, CL. Purification and structural analysis of a murine chemotactic cytokine (CP-10) with sequence homology to S100 proteins. *J Biol Chem.*, 1992 Apr 15, 267(11), 7499-504.

[163] Yang, Z; Tao, T; Raftery, MJ; Youssef, P; Di Girolamo, N; Geczy, CL. Proinflammatory properties of the human S100 protein S100A12. *J Leukoc Biol.*, 2001 Jun, 69(6), 986-94.

[164] Ryckman, C; Vandal, K; Rouleau, P; Talbot, M; Tessier, PA. Proinflammatory activities of S100: proteins S100A8, S100A9, and S100A8/A9 induce neutrophil chemotaxis and adhesion. *J Immunol.*, 2003 Mar 15, 170(6), 3233-42.

[165] Vandal, K; Rouleau, P; Boivin, A; Ryckman, C; Talbot, M; Tessier, PA. Blockade of S100A8 and S100A9 suppresses neutrophil migration in response to lipopolysaccharide. *J Immunol.* 2003 Sep 1, 171(5), 2602-9.

[166] Giorgi, R; Pagano, RL; Dias, MA; Aguiar-Passeti, T; Sorg, C; Mariano, M. Antinociceptive effect of the calcium-binding protein MRP-14 and the role played by neutrophils on the control of inflammatory pain. *J Leukoc Biol.*, 1998 Aug, 64(2), 214-20.

[167] Johne, B; Fagerhol, MK; Lyberg, T; Prydz, H; Brandtzaeg, P; Naess-Andresen, CF; et al. Functional and clinical aspects of the myelomonocyte protein calprotectin. *Mol Pathol.*, 1997 Jun, 50(3), 113-23.

[168] Murthy, AR; Lehrer, RI; Harwig, SS; Miyasaki, KT. In vitro candidastatic properties of the human neutrophil calprotectin complex. *J Immunol.*, 1993 Dec 1, 151(11), 6291-301.

[169] Sohnle, PG; Collins-Lech, C; Wiessner, JH. Antimicrobial activity of an abundant calcium-binding protein in the cytoplasm of human neutrophils. *J Infect Dis.*, 1991 Jan, 163(1), 187-92.

[170] Steinbakk, M; Naess-Andresen, CF; Lingaas, E; Dale, I; Brandtzaeg, P; Fagerhol, MK. Antimicrobial actions of calcium binding leucocyte L1 protein, calprotectin. *Lancet.*, 1990 Sep 29, 336(8718), 763-5.

[171] Yui, S; Mikami, M; Tsurumaki, K; Yamazaki, M. Growth-inhibitory and apoptosis-inducing activities of calprotectin derived from inflammatory exudate cells on normal fibroblasts: regulation by metal ions. *J Leukoc Biol.*, 1997 Jan, 61(1), 50-7.

[172] Foell, D; Frosch, M; Sorg, C; Roth, J. Phagocyte-specific calcium-binding S100 proteins as clinical laboratory markers of inflammation. *Clin Chim Acta.* 2004 Jun, 344(1-2), 37-51.

[173] Odink, K; Cerletti, N; Bruggen, J; Clerc, RG; Tarcsay, L; Zwadlo, G; et al. Two calcium-binding proteins in infiltrate macrophages of rheumatoid arthritis. *Nature.* 1987 Nov 5-11, 330(6143), 80-2.

[174] Zwadlo, G; Bruggen, J; Gerhards, G; Schlegel, R; Sorg, C. Two calcium-binding proteins associated with specific stages of myeloid cell differentiation are expressed by subsets of macrophages in inflammatory tissues. *Clin Exp Immunol.*, 1988 Jun, 72(3), 510-5.

[175] Foell, D; Wittkowski, H; Roth, J. Monitoring disease activity by stool analyses: from occult blood to molecular markers of intestinal inflammation and damage. *Gut.* 2009 Jun, 58(6), 859-68.

[176] Lugering, N; Stoll, R; Kucharzik, T; Schmid, KW; Rohlmann, G; Burmeister, G; et al. Immunohistochemical distribution and serum levels of the Ca(2+)-binding proteins MRP8, MRP14 and their heterodimeric form MRP8/14 in Crohn's disease. *Digestion.*, 1995, 56(5), 406-14.

[177] Lugering, N; Stoll, R; Schmid, KW; Kucharzik, T; Stein, H; Burmeister, G; et al. The myeloic related protein MRP8/14 (27E10 antigen)--usefulness as a potential marker for disease activity in ulcerative colitis and putative biological function. *Eur J Clin Invest.*, 1995 Sep, 25(9), 659-64.

[178] McCormick, MM; Rahimi, F; Bobryshev, YV; Gaus, K; Zreiqat, H; Cai, H; et al. S100A8 and S100A9 in human arterial wall. Implications for atherogenesis. *J Biol Chem.*, 2005 Dec 16, 280(50), 41521-9.

[179] Abe, J; Jibiki, T; Noma, S; Nakajima, T; Saito, H; Terai, M. Gene expression profiling of the effect of high-dose intravenous Ig in patients with Kawasaki disease. *J Immunol.*, 2005 May 1, 174(9), 5837-45.

[180] Rastaldi, MP; Ferrario, F; Crippa, A; Dell'Antonio, G; Casartelli, D; Grillo, C; et al. Glomerular monocyte-macrophage features in ANCA-positive renal vasculitis and cryoglobulinemic nephritis. *J Am Soc Nephrol.*, 2000 Nov, 11(11), 2036-43.

[181] Haga, HJ; Brun, JG; Berntzen, HB; Cervera, R; Khamashta, M; Hughes, GR. Calprotectin in patients with systemic lupus erythematosus: relation to clinical and laboratory parameters of disease activity. *Lupus.*, 1993 Feb, 2(1), 47-50.

[182] Kane, D; Roth, J; Frosch, M; Vogl, T; Bresnihan, B; FitzGerald, O. Increased perivascular synovial membrane expression of myeloid-related proteins in psoriatic arthritis. *Arthritis Rheum.*, 2003 Jun, 48(6), 1676-85.

[183] Youssef, P; Roth, J; Frosch, M; Costello, P; Fitzgerald, O; Sorg, C; et al. Expression of myeloid related proteins (MRP) 8 and 14 and the MRP8/14 heterodimer in rheumatoid arthritis synovial membrane. *J Rheumatol.*, 1999 Dec, 26(12), 2523-8.

[184] Vogl, T; Tenbrock, K; Ludwig, S; Leukert, N; Ehrhardt, C; van Zoelen, MA; et al. Mrp8 and Mrp14 are endogenous activators of Toll-like receptor 4, promoting lethal, endotoxin-induced shock. *Nat Med.*, 2007 Sep, 13(9), 1042-9.

[185] Beutler, B; Rietschel, ET. Innate immune sensing and its roots: the story of endotoxin. *Nat Rev Immunol.*, 2003 Feb, 3(2), 169-76.

[186] Clark, MA; Plank, LD; Connolly, AB; Streat, SJ; Hill, AA; Gupta, R; et al. Effect of a chimeric antibody to tumor necrosis factor-alpha on cytokine and physiologic responses in patients with severe sepsis--a randomized, clinical trial. *Crit Care Med.*, 1998 Oct, 26(10), 1650-9.

[187] Fisher, CJ; Jr., Agosti, JM; Opal, SM; Lowry, SF; Balk, RA; Sadoff, JC; et al. Treatment of septic shock with the tumor necrosis factor receptor:Fc fusion protein. The Soluble TNF Receptor Sepsis Study Group. *N Engl J Med.*, 1996 Jun 27, 334(26), 1697-702.

In: Sepsis: Symptoms, Diagnosis and Treatment
Editor: Joseph R. Brown, pp. 29-54

ISBN: 978-1-60876-609-3
© 2010 Nova Science Publishers, Inc.

Chapter 2

SEPSIS: ACUTE KIDNEY INJURY AND β_2-ADRENOCEPTOR THERAPY

*Akio Nakamura**

Department of Pediatrics, Teikyo University School of Medicine,
2-11-1, Kaga, Itabashi-ku, Tokyo, Japan 173-8605

ABSTRACT

Endotoxemia caused by Gram-negative bacteria can result in sepsis and organ dysfunction, which includes kidney injury and renal failure. The renal β_2-adrenoceptor (β_2-AR) system has an anti-inflammatory influence on the cytokine network during the course of immunologic responses. The previous reports indicated that the administration of β_2-AR agonists was found to attenuate the stimulation of renal TNF-α associated with lipopolysaccharide and Shiga toxin-2 of hemolytic uremic syndrome (HUS), which is considered to be a central mediator of the pathophysiologic changes. On the other hand, an altered expression and/or function of β_2-AR have been considered to be a pathogenetic factor in some disease states with inflammation; for example, heart failure and renal failure. These observations would suggest that blockade of functional β_2-AR activation might be associated with an increase risk for organ dysfunction following severe sepsis. In this chapter, we reviewed sepsis-induced renal injury and the genomic information to identify groups of patients with a high risk of developing sepsis-induced acute renal failure. In addition, we attempt to demonstrate a new insight into the immunological importance of β_2-AR activation in sepsis and an application of β_2-AR to septic renal failure and HUS. Furthermore, an *in vivo* β_2-AR gene therapy for the replacement of lost receptors as a consequence of sepsis was also described.

* Corresponding author: E-mail: akio@med. teikyo-u. ac. jp, FAX: 03-3579-8212, TEL: 03-3964-1211 (ext. 7077)

INTRODUCTION

According to the 1992 Consensus Conference on definitions for sepsis and organ failure, sepsis is defined as a systemic inflammatory response (SIRS) associated with infection (Figure 1). Sepsis leads to the excessive production of proinflammatory cytokines, which are considered to contribute to the development of organ failure and tissue inflammation [1, 2]. This response is especially pertinent in acute inflammatory diseases, such as acute renal failure (ARF), as inflammatory mediators can cause a dose-related reversible response in target endothelial cells.

There is a growing body of evidence that the β_2-adrenoceptor (β_2-AR) system has an anti-inflammatory influence on the cytokine network during the course of immunologic responses. For example, β_2-AR agonists inhibit the renal production of inflammatory cytokines, such as tumour necrosis factor (TNF-α). Moreover, the administration of β_2AR agonists is found to attenuate TNF-α gene expression associated with Shiga toxin (Stx) of hemolytic uremic syndrome (HUS) [3]. Recently, we demonstrated that the application of adenoviral mediated β_2-AR gene delivery to enhance renal β_2-AR activity affords the kidney protection against endotoxin-induced ARF [4]. These observations would suggest a possibility that a level of functional β_2-AR activation might decide an increase risk for renal dysfunction following severe sepsis. Therefore, increased understanding of the immunologic basis of β_2-AR function in the kidney provides important new information relevant to the treatment of ARF in inflammatory diseases and potential applications of β_2-AR gene therapy in renal damage and inflammation associated with sepsis.

SEPSIS-INDUCED RENAL INJURY

Acute Kidney Injury

Sepsis remains a worldwide problem and one that is associated with a high mortality rate. It is the leading cause of death in intensive care units (ICU) [5] and sepsis and its sequelae remains a major cause of ARF in both ICU and non-ICU [6]. ARF, recently renamed acute kidney injury (AKI), is a relatively frequent problem in patients with severe sepsis. Importantly, septic shock following surgery, trauma, burns, or severe infection was a common cause of ARF resulting in a high mortality rate [7]. It is recognized that severe sepsis results in excessive activation of inflammation and raised blood coagulation. In particular, endotoxemia caused by gram-negative bacteria can result in a systemic inflammatory response and organ dysfunction, which includes kidney ischemic and nephrotoxic damage [8, 9]. Pathological examination of the failing kidneys has revealed that inflammatory responses to sepsis resulted in the occurrence of focal necrosis of the proximal tubular epithelium, eosinophilic casts within proximal and distal tubules, and microthrombi in the glomerular capillaries [10]. Together these findings have implicated sepsis-induced inflammation, especially cytokines, in the pathogenesis of ARF.

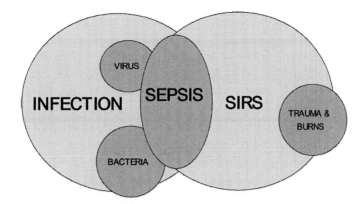

Figure 1. The definition of sepsis. Sepsis is defined as suspected or microbiologically proven infection together with SIRS.

Table 1. Positive association between sepsis with ARF or without ARF and polymorphisms

Genes	Allele	Illness/Ethnicity	Cases/Control subjects
TNF-α	TNF-α-308A	Sepsis/French whites	Septic shock/Healthy
		Septic shock	Survivors/non-Survivors
		ARF in neonate	ARF/non-ARF baby
		Post-operative sepsis/Taiwan Asian	Survivors/non-Survivors
		Dialysis-required ARF	Survivors/non-Survivors
TNF-β	TNF-β 252A homozygote	Post-operative sepsis/ German whites	Survivors/non-Survivors
IL-1ra	IL-raA2	Susceptibility to sepsis /German whites	Sepsis/Healthy
IL-6	IL-6-174C	ARF in neonate	ARF/non-ARF baby
IL-10	IL-10-592A	Sepsis	Survivors/non-Survivors
	IL-10-1082G	Dialysis-required ARF	Survivors/non-Survivors
HSP	HSP70-2+1267GG	ARF in neonate	ARF/non-ARF baby
	HSP70-2+1267AA	Septic shock	Sepsis/non-Sepsis
TLR4	Asp299Gly	Septic shock	Survivors/non-Survivors
		Septic shock	Septic shock/Healthy
CD14	CD14-159T	Septic shock/French whites	Sepsis/Healthy
		Septic shock/French whites	Survivors/non-Survivors

ARF:acute renal failure, HSP:heat shock protein, TLR:toll-like receptor.

Role of Cytokines in ARF

The role of pro-inflammatory cytokines in the development of endotoxin-mediated ARF has been increasingly recognized [11, 12]. TNF-α is a cytokine that initiates the inflammatory cascade that induces the production of numerous additional mediators associated with endothelial and tissue injury which comprise the multiple organ dysfunction syndrome [13-15]. Similarly, interleukin-10 (IL-10) is an important component of the anti-inflammatory cytokine network in sepsis which suppresses gene expression and synthesis of pro-inflammatory cytokines, such as TNF- α [16, 17]. These observations suggest that the balance between pro- and anti-inflammatory mediators plays an important role in the initiation and regulation of host inflammatory responses that determine the severity of acute illnesses such as ARF. Importantly, cytokines such as TNF- α, IL-1, IL-6, and IL-10 affect renal function in a variety of different ways [18]. High levels of these cytokines induce systemic hypotension which can lead to renal hypoperfusion; they directly influence renal hemodynamics by damaging glomerular endothelial and mesangial cells; they may induce the release and promote the effect of vasoactive mediators, such as endothelin, prostaglandins, and nitric oxide [19, 20]; finally, they may play a role in the initiation and progression of certain risk factors for ARF. In sepsis, cytokine release results in leukocyte activation along with the expression of adhesion molecules, oxygen-free radicals, arachidonic acid metabolites, platelet-activating factor, nitric oxide, endothelins, and heat shock proteins (HSP) [21,22]. Thus, it is this cytokine cascade that contributes to endothelial cell damage of the renal vasculature, leading to the development of ARF. Moreover, bacterial products can activate neutrophils within an already injured kidney [23], with IL-8 acting to recruit neutrophils to sites of inflammation [24]. Recently, human activated protein C, an endogenous protein that inhibits thrombosis and inflammation, decreased the relative risk of death in patients with severe sepsis [25]. However, it remains unclear which group of patients with sepsis benefit most from this therapy. Investigation into the specific genetic makeup may not only predict the risk of sepsis but may also to the development of organ dysfunction or ultimately death.

The Risk of ARF and Polymorphisms

Several studies have provided evidence supporting the view that genetic polymorphisms of cytokine-encoding genes can contribute to individual variance in inflammatory responses and they have postulated an association with risk for cytokine-mediated disorders, such as ARF (Table 1). It has been recognized that allelic polymorphisms in the promoter regions of cytokine genes regulate the expression of cytokines and may be of functional relevance. In particular, polymorphisms involving the promoter (5'-flanking) region of the TNF-α and IL-10 genes may affect transcriptional activity and thereby influence outcome in critically ill patients with ARF who require dialysis [26]. It has been reported that mortality is significantly higher in patients with the -308 G→A polymorphism in the promoter region of the TNF-α gene, which was associated with higher levels of TNF-α production, and the -1082 G→A polymorphism of the promoter region of the IL-10 gene, associated with lower levels of IL-10 production [26]. HSP72 plays a fundamental role in the ischemic tolerance of immature kidneys and protects premature babies against hypoxic renal injury [27, 28]. Fekete *et al* [27] indicated that in low birth weight neonates carrying the HSP72 +1267GG genetic variation, which is associated with lower levels of HSP72 production, the risk of ARF was increased. Furthermore, they found that ARF risk was directly associated with high TNF-α producer and low IL-6 producer genotypes in preterm neonates [29]. On the other hand, several studies have found an association between the risk of sepsis and polymorphism of genes involved with the immune response genes; TNF-β gene variant [30], IL-1Ra allele-2 [31], IL-6-174C allele [32], IL-10-592A [33], CD14-159T [34], HSP70+2267AA [35], Toll like receptor(TLR)-4 Asp299Gly [36]. Polymorphism in these genes has been studied extensively and has been associated with adverse clinical outcomes among patients suffering from sepsis. However, these polymorphisms play in modulating susceptibility to or severity of ARF has not been investigated in sufficient depth to date.

IMMUNOLOGIC EFFECTS OF β$_2$-AR

Modulation of Immune Function

Sepsis involves activation of both the immune and the neuroendocrine systems. The modulation of immune function by catecholamines is pleiotypic and affects a range of cells in the immune system, including T cells, B cells, and NK cells [37]. In response to stress, norepinephrine and the related sympathetic catecholamine epinephrine are released into the blood-stream and in vitro they have been shown to alter several aspects of lymphocyte function, including inhibition of proliferation and differentiation [38], apoptosis [39], and interferon production in Th1 cells [40].

The β$_2$-ARs are distributed widely in vascular tissue and are the primary adrenergic receptor causing vasodilatation upon stimulation with endogenous catecholamines [41-43]. Furthermore, β$_2$-ARs are present on lymphocytes and are involved with the regulation of the immune responses. There is increasing evidence that activation of β$_2$-ARs can modulate the production of pro- and anti-inflammatory cytokines, such as TNF, IL-1, IL-6, IL-10, IL-12, in some tissues and organs [44-47]. We also demonstrated that in renal resident macrophage cells, the glomerular mesangial cells, and tubular epithelial cells and in brain astrocyte cells, the administration of β$_2$-AR agonists modulated the production and gene expression of TNF-α and IL-6 [45, 48]. An altered expression and function of the β$_2$-AR signal transduction mechanism in an organ is involved in the uncontrolled immune response that occurs during sepsis.

Anti-Inflammatory Effects in Sepsis

Bernardin et al [49] showed that the activation of adenylate cyclase by β$_2$-AR was heterogeneously desensitized in peripheral blood mononuclear cells freshly isolated from septic patients. These observations would be compatible with the suggestion that abnormalities in the β$_2$-adrenergic control of organ function could be implicated in the pathogenesis of septic shock. β$_2$-AR agonists have been demonstrated to reduce both the increased permeability and the production of inflammatory mediators from endothelial cells [50, 51] and to prevent organ and tissue damage in response to an endotoxin challenge [3, 4]. Tighe et al [52] have shown experimentally that in a porcine faecal peritonitis model of multi-organ failure, the administration of β_2-AR agonists reduces hepatic cellular injury during sepsis. Conversely, the β_2-AR antagonist, ICI 118551, enhanced the hepatic injury normally found during sepsis in the porcine model. These findings were supported by another report in which the β_2-AR agonist terbutaline was shown to attenuate the product of inflammatory cytokine mediators in the lungs and liver of sheep during endotoxic shock [30, 53]. On the other hand, in the kidney, it was found that the activation of β_2-ARs attenuated the production of TNF-α [4, 47] and suppressed kidney damage associated with the endotoxemia [54] and similarly the Stx-2 which causes HUS [3]. Endotoxin not only stimulates the production of cytokines but also the production of other mediators, such as histamine, leukotriene C and D, and prostaglandin D in human tissues. Importantly, β_2-AR agonists are able to suppress production of these mediators as well as cytokines [50, 55, 56]. Moreover, high levels of cyclic adenosine monophosphate (cAMP) in neutrophils caused by exposure to β_2-AR agonists can inhibit the generation of oxygen radicals [57]. It was further reported that a high level of cAMP in the endothelial cells was able to inhibit several key enzymes in the inflammatory pathway, leading to a reduced release of inflammatory mediators such as platelet-activating factor, histamine, and arachidonic acid derivatives [58]. Recent experiments indicated that the use of β_2-AR agonists had beneficial actions in chronic inflammatory diseases, including multiple sclerosis [59], rheumatoid arthritis [60], and hepatitis [61].

Intracellular Mechanisms

Intracellular signaling following β_2-AR activation is largely effected through a cAMP and protein kinase A (PKA) pathway. β_2-AR agonists activate their trimeric G protein-linked receptors to produce the stimulatory G protein (Gs) which stimulates adenylate cyclase to form cAMP and activate PKA. In the respiratory tract, cAMP induces airway relaxation through phosphorylation of muscle regulatory proteins and attenuation of cellular Ca^{2+} concentrations. Alternative cAMP-independent pathways have also been described involving activation of membrane maxi-K^+ channels and coupling through the inhibitory G protein (Gi) to the mitogen-activated protein kinase (MAPK) system.

The intracellular mechanisms by which activation of β_2-ARs inhibit inflammatory mediators has been examined by Tighe et al [51]. In this study, they indicated that cAMP-PKA activation was involved in activating gene transcription agents to produce anti-inflammatory proteins such as IL-10. Moreover, PKA inhibited phospholipase C and MAPK to determine the production of pro-inflammatory cytokines. Additionally, van der Poll et al [62] indicated that pre-exposure of healthy humans to a constant infusion of epinephrine before injection of endotoxin attenuates the production of the pro-inflammatory cytokine TNF-α and simultaneously potentiates the production of the anti-inflammatory cytokine IL-10 through the adenylate cyclase-cAMP-PKA pathway [63, 64]. Furthermore, Panina-Bordignon et al. [65] presented evidence that β_2-AR agonists inhibited IL-12 production by human monocytes in response to lipopolysaccharide (LPS). The β_2-AR mediated inhibition of IL-12 correlated with β_2-AR stimulation and with increased levels of intracellular cAMP. Taken together, it is recognized that the cAMP-PKA pathway plays a critical role in the regulation of inflammatory cytokine production via β_2-AR activation.

KIDNEY AND β_2-AR SYSTEM

β_2-AR

β-AR belongs to a large family of the G-protein-coupled receptors that are characterized by seven transmembrane helices. Three subtypes of β-ARs (β_1-AR, β_2-AR, β_3-AR) are detected in the mammalian tissues. Molecular biological cloning approaches showed that β_2-AR gene is an intronless single gene coding 413 amino acid and is located on chromosome 5q31-33. β_2-ARs are involved in fundamental processes such as cell growth, differentiation, and metabolism and play important roles in cardiovascular, respiratory, metabolic, reproductive and central nervous system functions (Table 2). The β_2-ARs are found throughout the body including the heart, lung, blood vessels, lymphocyte and kidneys. In the heart, β_2-ARs have been localized to the ventricular walls where they primarily determine ventricular contractility. In the respiratory tract, the β_2-ARs are the predominant subtype in all segments but the β_2-AR-mediated adenylate cyclase response is tissue-dependent, with higher activity being present in the tracheal membranes than the bronchial or pulmonary segments. The β_2-ARs are also distributed widely in vascular tissue and are the primary adrenergic receptor causing vasodilatation upon stimulation with endogenous catecholamines. In clinical medicine, β_2-AR agonists are standard agents in the treatment of bronchial asthma and chronic bronchitis. A majority of β_2-AR agonists is eliminated via the kidneys as an unchanged substance. It is likely that such agents will exert pharmacological effects during their passage through the nephron. However, these pharmacological effects have, to our knowledge, not been taken into consideration when using these compounds in clinical practice because a role of β_2-AR in the regulation of renal function remains unclear.

Renal β_2-AR Pharmacology

The β-ARs are located in the kidneys [66-68] and the receptors are known to participate in the regulation of glomerular filtration rate (GFR), sodium reabsorption, acid-base balance and renin secretion [69]. Immunoreactivity for β_1-ARs was found in mesangial cells, juxtaglomerular granular cells, the macula densa epithelium, proximal and distal tubular segments, and acid-secreting type A intercalated cells of the cortical and medullary collecting ducts. On the other hand, β_2-ARs were predominantly localized in the apical and subapical compartment of proximal and, to a lesser extent, distal tubular epithelia [69]. This anatomic location provides evidence for a role of β_2-ARs in the control of renal tubular function. It has been reported that β_2-AR activation enhances sodium reabsorption through increased renal epithelial sodium channel (ENaC) activity [70-72]. In addition, the presence of functional β_2-

AR in cultured rat proximal tubule epithelial cells was demonstrated by the observation that β_2-AR activation resulted in increases in Sodium-Potassium-adenosine triphosphatase (Na-K-ATPase) activity and transcellular sodium transport as a consequence of increased apical sodium entry [73]. Furthermore, Singh and Linas[74] found that β_2-AR-mediated increases in Na-K-ATPase activity and sodium flux were transduced by protein kinase C (PKC), not PKA, acting to increase apical Na entry. In an *in vivo* study, Hashimoto *et al* [75] indicated that β_2-AR activation produced a decrease in urine flow, free water and osmolar clearance and also excretion of electrolytes in rat and dog renal tubules. In addition, they showed that renal blood flow and GFR were reduced by β_2-AR agonists with the concomitant fall of systemic blood pressure [75]. Boivin *et al* [69] reported that there was a high density of β_2-ARs in the membranes of smooth muscle cells from renal arteries. Administration of β_2-AR agonists had no effect on blood coagulation or hemolysis but inhibited the edema and increase in permeability of blood vessels induced by acetic acid [75]. Thus, the β_2- adrenergic system has the ability to modulate both the renal vasculature and renal tubule solute and water transport.

Table 2. Effects of β_2 adrenoceptor agonist

System	adrenoceptor type	Response to stimulation
Heart	$\beta1$ $\beta2$	Tachycardia
	$\beta1$	Contraction
Bronchus	$\beta2$	Dilatation
Brain	$\beta1$ $\beta2$	?
Gut	$\beta1$	Relaxation
	$\beta3$	
Metabolism	$\beta2$	Inhibition (Insulin secretion)
	$\beta3$	Lipolysis
Vessel	$\beta1$	Dilatation (Coronary arteries)
	$\beta2$	Dilatation (Renal arteries)
Kidney	$\beta1$	Stimulation (Renin secretion)
	$\beta2$	Sodium reabsorption

Defense Mechanisms for Septic ARF

(1) Inhibition of renal TNF-α production

In many types of renal glomerulonephritis, macrophages infiltrate into the glomerulus and interstitium and this has been taken as being the initial step in inducing renal damage [76]. Furthermore, it has been reported that macrophages are involved in the development of interstitial nephritis and obstructive uropathy [77]. Although the mechanisms mediating the macrophage-induced renal damage remains unclear, the pathophysiological developments in these renal diseases are associated with raised TNF-α [76] which plays a role in ischemic and toxic chemical injury within renal tissue [78]. Thus, there is a strong possibility that renal TNF-α generation is one of the most important factors in the pathophysiology of renal disease and injury. Previous investigators [47] have reported that elevation of intracellular cAMP is associated with the suppression of macrophage activation and cytokine production. Our own studies in the kidney also demonstrated that activation of the cAMP signaling pathway by means of β_2-AR agonists down-regulated TNF-α gene expression using renal resident macrophage cells exposed to endotoxin[80]. Consequently, the renal β_2-AR system was able to modify the inflammatory responses initiated in sepsis-induced renal injury through the inhibition of renal TNF-α generation.

(2) Modulation of IL-6

Amongst these pro-inflammatory cytokines, IL-6 is a pleiotropic cytokine which is involved in inflammatory and immune responses, acute phase reactions and hematopoiesis. At the level of the kidney, IL-6 is a key factor in mediating various components of the immune and inflammatory response [81]. There is increasing evidence that activation of β_2-ARs can modulate the production of LPS-induced inflammatory cytokines. However, the action of β_2-AR stimulation on IL-6 production is quite controversial. Liao et al [46] observed that β_2-AR mediated processes increased LPS-induced IL-6 production in liver cells, while Maimone et al [82] reported that exposure of astrocytes to norepinephrine elevated IL-6 which was mediated predominantly by β_2-AR and the activation of adenylate cyclase. It is recognized that intracellular cAMP plays an important role in the stimulation of IL-6 gene expression [83] and it has been suggested that raised IL-6 production due to β_2-AR activation is mediated through the cAMP pathway. On the other hand, Straub et al. [84] demonstrated that isoproterenol inhibited IL-6 secretion in the spleen, while our own studies also indicated an inhibitory effect of β_2-AR activation following LPS-induced IL-6 gene transcription in rat astrocytes [85]. Furthermore, in an in vivo study, epinephrine infusion into human subjects did not affect IL-6 production following an LPS challenge [62]. These findings suggest that factors and/or regulatory mechanisms other than the cAMP pathway contribute to β_2-AR mediated IL-6 production. Therefore, using renal resident macrophage cells treated with endotoxin, LPS, and β_2-AR agonist, terbutaline, we investigated the intracellular mechanisms in up-regulating or down-regulating IL-6 production [70].

The results from this experiment, terbutaline at high concentrations (10^{-6}M) significantly up-regulated IL-6 by approximately 25% (P < 0. 05), whereas at a lower concentration (10^{-8}M), it down-regulated IL-6 production by 42% (P < 0. 05). Terbutaline (10^{-8}M and 10^{-6} M) caused a concentration and time-dependent stimulation of cAMP (P<0. 05) and a time-dependent decrease in MAPK activity (P<0. 05) and TNF- α production (P<0. 05). Following the addition of a cAMP inhibitor, IL-6 promoter activity was correlated with TNF- α levels and MAPK activity. The terbutaline-induced down-regulation of IL-6 gene production was mediated by an inhibitory effect of terbutaline on TNF-α, which was exerted through the MAPK and cAMP pathways, whereas the up-regulation appeared to be due to a direct action of intracellular cAMP. Therefore, the modulation of endotoxin-induced IL-6 levels by β_2-ARs depends on the balance between a direct effect of cAMP as a stimulator of IL-6 and an indirect action of TNF- α as a suppresser of IL-6 through cAMP and/or MAPK (p42/p44) pathways.

(3) Inhibition of apoptosis

HUS is characterized by renal failure, thrombocytopenia and hemolytic anemia and is often induced by Stx producing strains of *Escherichia coli* [86, 87]. The most extensive tissue damage in HUS occurs in the kidney and reports have indicated that renal tubular impairment is a contributor to the development of HUS [88, 89]. Stx induces an apoptotic signal transduction cascade associated with enhanced expression of Bax in epithelial cells and the Stx-stimulated cell death was blocked by overexpression of Bcl-2 [90, 91]. Zhu et al [92] observed that the β_2-AR agonist, clenbuterol, not only increased Bcl-2 expression but also decreased Bax expression in a rat model of forebrain ischemia. These findings suggested the possibility that β_2-AR activation could have a major anti-apoptotic action. To provide further support for this view, we investigated the molecular mechanisms underlying the action of β_2-AR stimulation on Stx-induced apoptosis [93]. Apoptosis is regulated by several pathways, such as caspases, MAPK and cAMP-PKA cascade. This experiment focused on the effect of β_2-AR activation on Stx2-induced apoptosis in renal tubular cells and the contribution of these signaling pathways.

Cultured human adenocarcinoma-derived renal tubular cells (ACHN) were exposed to Stx (64 pg/mL) for 2–24 hr following the addition of the β_2-AR agonist (terbutaline) to the incubation medium. Stx-induced apoptosis and its amelioration by β_2-AR activation was confirmed using DNA degradation assays and by flow cytometry for annexin V, mitochondrial membrane potential and caspase (-3 and -7) activity. Exposure of cells to Stx for 24 hr increased the DNA fragmentation to 11. 6±0. 9%, compared to 3. 3±0. 2% in control cells (*P*<0. 05) but was decreased to approximately 5–7% (*P*<0. 05) in the presence of terbutaline. Furthermore, Stx-stimulated apoptosis, detected by TUNEL, annexin V and mitochondrial potential, was inhibited by terbutaline (*P*<0. 05) which was prevented by cAMP-PKA inhibitors and a β_2-AR antagonist. However, inhibition of Stx-mediated caspase activity by terbutaline was partially blocked by cAMP-PKA inhibitors. On the other hand, p38MAPK inhibition by terbutaline prevented Stx-induced apoptosis and caspase activity through a cAMP-independent pathway via β_2-AR. These data indicate that β_2-AR activation can inhibit Stx-induced apoptosis of the cells, which may be caused by a reduction in caspase activity through cAMP-PKA activation and the p38MAPK pathway (Figure 2).

(4) Modulation of innate immunity

LPS is sensed by LPS-binding protein (LBP), CD14, and toll-like receptor 4 (TLR4). CD14/ TLR4 complexes are the primary signaling receptor for gram-negative bacterial LPS [94]. When presented to CD14 by LBP, LPS is delivered to high-affinity transmembrane receptor such as TLR4 [95], leading to production of TNF-α [96]. Thus, CD14 and TLR4 are critical for LPS-mediated production of TNF-α. Injection of LPS reproduces many of the manifestations of sepsis and organ dysfunction, including kidney damage and renal failure [9]. The pathological mechanisms responsible for this renal dysfunction involve several mediators, and an important class is the early proinflammatory cytokines, such as TNF-α [78, 79]. Cunningham et al. [97] have showed that mice deficient in tumour necrosis factor receptor 1 (TNFR1) are resistant to LPS-induced ARF, and that TNFR1 mediates LPS-induced ARF within the kidney. Therefore, these evidences suggest a possibility that activation of β_2-AR signaling pathway could attenuate renal TNF-α production through CD14 and TLR4-dependent mechanisms, which, in turn, contributes to the protection against LPS-induced ARF. Recently, we clarified the importance of functional β_2-AR in regulating innate immunity in LPS-induced ARF [98]. In the animal experiment, rats were challenged with LPS, and the role of β_2-AR-mediated intrarenal cAMP in the regulation of CD14-TLR4-TNF-α signaling pathway in the kidney was determined using co-administration with β_2-AR antagonist ICI118, 551.

Figure 2 depicts these findings and summarizes the known effects of LPS and Stx and the possible interaction with β_2-AR signaling pathway.

STRATEGY FOR SEPTIC ARF

β_2-AR Agonists

(1) Endotoxin-induced sepsis

Cytokines play an important role in pathogenesis of endotoxin-induced ARF. Some studies indicated that β_2-AR activation regulated TNF-α and IL-6 production in cultured cells stimulated by endotoxin. In liver cells, Liao et al. [46] documented that β_2-AR -mediated processes were able to regulate TNF-α and IL-6 production. Severn et al. [47] demonstrated suppression of TNF-α production by isoproterenol in cultured human blood cells stimulated by LPS, which was mediated by increased intracellular cAMP levels. Hetier et al. [48] investigated the regulation of TNF-α gene expression in the microglia cells upon stimulation with LPS, and observed that isoproterenol, via an action at β_2-AR, was able to influence the regulatory processes of TNF-α gene expression. In the kidney, we have reported that LPS-stimulated TNF-α and IL-6 gene transcription, mRNA accumulation and protein levels were suppressed by β_2-AR activation with terbutaline using cultured renal resident macrophage cells [80] and mesangial cells [45,99].

There is also in vivo evidence that β_2-AR agonists can modulate the production of TNF-α and IL-6 in some tissues and organs under the state of endotoxemia. Previously, we investigated whether, in vivo, the administration of β_2-AR agonists regulate renal TNF-α and IL-6 mRNA following LPS stimulation to cause endotoxaemia [100]. In this experiment, 4-week-old Wistar rats pre-treated with the β_2-AR agonist terbutaline or formoterol, and/or the β-AR and β_2-AR antagonists (propanolol, ICI118,551), were injected with LPS (1 mg i. p.), and then 2, 4 or 6 h later, kidneys (cortex, medulla), spleen, thymus and plasma were assayed TNF-α and IL-6 mRNA levels and their respective protein release. The results indicated that administration of β_2-AR agonists suppressed TNF- α mRNA expression in the whole kidney, by 61% ($P<0.05$), as well as plasma, spleen and thymus TNF- α protein and mRNA expression 2 h after injection of LPS. On the other hand, although IL-6 levels in plasma, spleen and thymus mRNA expression were suppressed significantly by administration of β_2-AR agonists, the basal- and LPS-induced IL-6 mRNA levels in the whole kidney were increased 1.6- and 1.2-fold ($P<0.05$), respectively, by treatment with β_2-AR agonists. These findings suggest the existence of tissue specific regulation of IL-6 production in the kidney by β_2-AR activation.

(2) HUS

As described previously, Stx-producing *Escherichia coli* are responsible for some cases of HUS [86, 87]. There are two forms of Stx and they are also known as verocytotoxins, Stx1 and Stx2. It has been reported that induction of the globotriaosyleramide (Gb3) receptor, known to be the functional receptor for Stx, is one mechanism by which inflammatory mediators increase susceptibility to Stx [101]. The major pathogenesis of HUS has been ascribed to initial endothelial and vascular damage. However, evidence has been reported from some studies in human, of primary renal tubular cell damage in HUS [89]. The receptor sites for Stx binding in normal kidney sections are most prominent in renal cortical tubules [89,102], probably in the distal tubule. Renal biopsy studies early in the course of HUS have suggested a direct action on the proximal tubules while cultured epithelial cells from this region express very high levels of Gb3 [90,103]. These reports imply that renal tubular impairment contributes to the development of HUS.

Exposure of renal tubular epithelial cells to Stx causes cytotoxicity, and the potency of this toxin is enhanced in the presence of TNF- α [88]. It has been shown that Stx induces TNF- α production and that activation of β_2-ARs downregulates TNF- α. However, little was known about the signaling pathway by which β_2-AR agonists suppress the Stx-induced TNF- α gene transcription in the renal tubular cells. Previously, we investigated that the possible signaling components involved in this pathway [3]. In this experiment, MAPK, activating protein-1 (AP-1), and nuclear factor-κB (NFκ-B) were measured to evaluate the regulatory mechanisms involved in TNF- α gene transcription in ACHN exposed to Stx in the presence or absence of a β_2-AR agonist. Stx (4 pg/ml) stimulated MAPK (p42/p44, p38) and AP-1 and increased TNF- α promoter activity by 2.4-fold. The increase in TNF- α was attenuated by both a p42/p44 inhibitor, PD098059 (10^{-6} M), and a p38 inhibitor, SB203580 (10^{-6} M), and AP-1—binding activity was inhibited by PD098059. Terbutaline (10^{-6} M to 10^{-8} M) suppressed MAPK (p42/p44, p38), NF-κB (p50, p65), and TNF-α promoter activity in a dose-dependent way that was prevented by the β_2-AR antagonist, ICI118,551. However, inhibition of MAPK (p42/p44) and TNF-α promoter activity was partially prevented by the cAMP-protein kinase (PKA) inhibitors, H-89 (5 x 10^{-6} M) and KT5720 (10^{-5} M), whereas the suppression of p38 MAPK or NF-κB (p50) was not blocked by these inhibitors. The suppression of NF-κB (p65) was completely overcome by H-89 or KT5720. Consequently, the downregulation of TNF-α transcription by terbutaline was mediated by an inhibitory effect of β_2-AR activation on MAPK (p42/p44, p38) and NF-κB p50/p65), which were exerted through a cAMP-PKA pathway and a cAMP-independent mechanism (Figure 2).

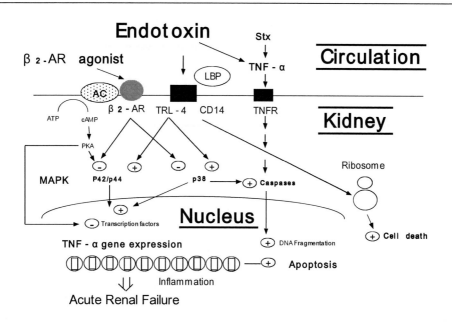

Figure 2. Proposed model of pathways mediating TNF-α production and apoptosis in renal cells exposed to endotoxin, Stx and/or β_2-adrenoceptor (β_2-AR) agonists. Endotoxin sensed by LBP initiates intracellular signaling events via CD14 and TLR-4 in the kidney. The CD14 and TLR-4 complexes could result in the stimulation of renal TNF-α production through the activation of transcription factors (AP-1, NF-κB) via MAPK signaling cascades. Stx also stimulates TNF-α gene expression through these signaling cascades and activated caspase cascade (caspase-3), thereby signaling cells to undergo apoptosis. On the other hand, β_2-ARs couple to adenylate cyclases (AC) to raise intracellular level of cAMP-PKA, which inhibits TLR4-CD14-TNF-α signaling cascades, p42/p44 MAPK and caspases activation. Moreover, β_2-AR activation suppresses p38 MAPK activity with subsequent caspase-3 inhibition through a cAMP-independent mechanism. Importantly, β_2-AR activation inhibits the renal TNF-α–induced inflammation and apoptosis associated with endotoxin and Stx, which, in turn, could result in ARF.
+: activation, - :inhibition.

β_2-AR Gene Therapy

(1) Contribution of β_2-AR gene delivery to renal physiology

For the purpose of activation and restoration of β_2-AR function, drugs targeting β_2-AR signaling, including β_2-AR agonists, may be used as a first-line approach for therapy. However, administration of β_2-AR agonists to regulate β_2-AR function has an inherently limited efficacy, partly because of the down-regulation and desensitization of β_2-ARs [99]. On the other hand, in vivo gene therapy using adenoviral constructs containing the β_2-AR gene has been demonstrated to be an efficient and reproducible global transgene delivery system which results in long term expression in the organ as has been reported in the myocardium [105]. Therefore, the application of adenoviral mediated β_2-AR gene delivery to elevate β_2-AR density and prevent desensitization would be an attractive option whereby β_2-ARs could be active over a prolonged period. With this in mind we utilized adenoviral-mediated β_2-AR gene delivery to investigate whether over-expression of β_2-AR could alter both biochemical and *in vivo* renal function and to test the hypothesis that the β_2-AR gene delivery affords the kidney protection against endotoxin-induced ARF [4]. As a construction of recombinant adenovirus, the human β_2-AR expressing adenovirus (Adeno-β_2-AR) and the cytoplasmic β-galactosidase expressing adenovirus (Adeno-LacZ) as a control were used in the study. These adenoviruses were a replication-deficient first-generation type V adenovirus with deletions of the E1 gene (Figure 3). These viruses were injected into the right kidney of rats using a 25-gauge needle attached to a 1ml syringe.

To test how long β_2-AR transgene over expression was supported in the renal tissue, β-AR density levels were measured in the right and left kidneys during a 5 wk period after intraparenchymal gene delivery. There was a sharp increase in β-AR density level 2 wks after intraparenchymal Adeno-β_2-AR gene delivery (10^9 total viral particles:t. v. p) in the right kidney, which was sustained until the 4 wk time-point. Furthermore, measurable β-AR over expression was also observed in the contra-lateral left kidney, which was elevated at 2 wks after the gene delivery. β-AR density in the right and left kidneys after intraparenchymal Adeno- LacZ gene delivery (10^9 t. v. p) was unaltered over this timeframe.

The time course of glomerular filtration rate (GFR :ml/min/100g body weight) after delivery of various doses of Adeno-β_2-AR was investigated. Although there was a significant increase (P<0. 05) in GFR 2wks after intraparenchymal delivery of Adeno-β_2-AR (10^9t. v. p), GFR levels at 1, 3, and 4wks after delivery of Adeno-β_2-AR (10^{8-9}t. v. p) were not changed compared to those in Adeno- LacZ treated rats. In contrast, the higher dose of 10^{10}t. v. p Adeno-β_2-AR produced a diminished GFR with advancing age. The changes in time course of FENa or FEK (%) following various doses of Adeno-β_2-AR were also measured over this timeframe. There was a significant decrease in FENa (P<0.05) 1-2wks after intraparenchymal delivery of Adeno-β_2-AR(10^{8-9}t. v. p), while at 3 and 4wks after delivery of Adeno-β_2-AR (10^{8-9}t. v. p) it was not different from that in Adeno- LacZ treated rats. FEK levels after delivery of Adeno-β_2-AR (10^{8-9}t. v. p) were unchanged compared to those in Adeno- LacZ treated rats while there was a significant increase in FEK 3-4wks after intraparenchymal delivery of the higher dose of Adeno-β_2-AR (10^{10}t. v. p). These results indicated that GFR, FENa, and FEK became stable approximately 3-4 wks after the delivery of Adeno-β_2-AR (10^{8-9}t. v. p). Furthermore, Adeno- β_2-AR (10^9 t. v. p) did not change weight, Blood Pressure (BP) or Heart Rate compared with those of physiological saline (PBS) treated rats without adenovirus delivery. This suggested the safety of Adeno- β_2-AR (10^9 t. v. p) delivery

(2) Effects of β_2-AR gene therapy on septic ARF

These effects were investigated using intraperitoneal injection of LPS (5mg/kg) to induce renal failure in control and Adeno-β_2-AR treated rats. Control rats of this experiment were injected intraperitoneally with an equal volume of PBS. The β_2-AR antagonist ICI 118,551 was given intraperitoneally 2 h before an injection of the LPS or PBS. The experiment was performed on the 25th day after the delivery of 10^9 t. v. p of Adeno-β_2-AR, which was chosen as the therapeutic dose [4]. It can be seen in Figure 4 that GFR in the Adeno-β_2-AR treated rats was not changed 24h after the injection of LPS while in the control rats it was significantly (P<0. 05) depressed by the LPS challenge. The addition of the antagonist, ICI 118,551 blocked the ability of the Adeno-β_2-AR treated rats to maintain GFR, suggesting that constitutive β_2-AR activity plays an important role in preserving renal function against the endotoxin. Figure 5 indicated that β_2–AR density measured in the right kidney from control rats was significantly (P<0. 05) depressed 24 h after the LPS challenge. The renal β_2–AR density in Adeno-β_2–AR treated rats, although higher than the control rats, was also decreased by the injection of LPS (P<0. 05). Besides kidney, the lung β_2–AR levels were also depressed by the treatments with LPS (Figure 5). On the other hand, renal cAMP content (of both right and left kidneys) was depressed (P<0. 05) by the LPS challenge in the control rats but not in the Adeno-β_2–AR treated rats. The responses in renal cAMP level induced by the LPS in both groups correlated with the changes in renal β–AR density.

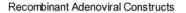

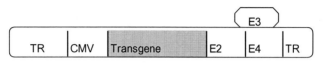

Recombinant Adenoviral Constructs

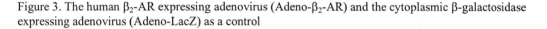

Transgene	Adenovirus
Human β_2-AR	Adeno-β_2-AR
β-galactosidase	Adeno-LacZ

Figure 3. The human β_2-AR expressing adenovirus (Adeno-β_2-AR) and the cytoplasmic β-galactosidase expressing adenovirus (Adeno-LacZ) as a control

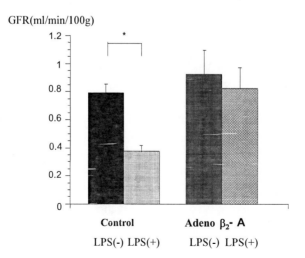

Figure 4. Rescue of endotoxin-induced renal dysfunction in the Adeno-β_2-AR rats. GFR (ml/min per 100 g body weight) levels in rats treated with PBS (control) or Adeno-β_2-AR were estimated 24h after LPS (5 mg/kg intraperitoneally) injection. Data are mean ± SE. *P<0. 05 *versus* PBS or Adeno-β_2-AR rats without LPS treatment. n = 5 to 8.

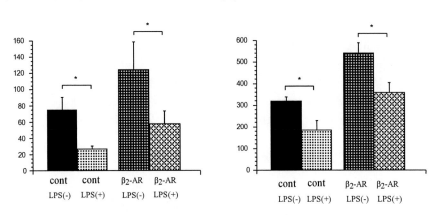

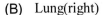

β2-adrenoceptor density
(f mol/mg membrane protein)

Figure 5. β_2-AR density levels of the right kidney(A) and the right lung (B) in rats treated with PBS (control) or Adeno-β_2-AR were estimated 24h after LPS (5 mg/kg intraperitoneally) injection. Data are mean ± SE. *P<0. 05 *versus* PBS or Adeno-β_2-AR rats without LPS treatment. n =6 to 8.

From these findings, we found that renal over expression of β_2–ARs using gene transfer with Adeno-β_2–AR was effective in preventing endotoxin-induced renal injury. This finding was intriguing in that the sepsis induced renal failure occurred with the decreases in β_2-AR density and cAMP activity, which suggested an impaired renal β_2–AR signaling system. Thus, the delivery of Adeno-β_2-AR gene could be a potential novel therapeutic strategy for treatment of ARF associated with sepsis. It is likely that this protective effect of β_2-AR activation is exerted through the intracellular cAMP-PKA pathway as previous studies reported found that cAMP-PKA activation was necessary to prevent the development of ARF [106]. Indeed, it was reported that the fall in renal cAMP level was correlated with the depression in GFR caused by the LPS challenge [107].

(3) Optional route of administration and safety

In clinical trials with adenoviral vectors, route-dependent efficacy of gene therapy has been a significant concern [108]. Generally, the direct injection into the target organ is more efficacious than systemic administration, via intravenous or intramuscular routes. However, gene therapy aimed to overcome systemic inflammation, for example as occurs in sepsis, requires a suitable injection route for the viral gene vector, such that it can effectively incorporate into the major target organs of sepsis, the kidney, lung, liver, and heart. An additional consideration of gene therapy using adenoviral vectors is the potential toxicity, which may cause inflammation on the tissues [109]. Therefore, high transduction rates, bio-safety of the gene product and minimally invasive administration are required to ensure an optimal route of gene delivery for a successful therapeutic strategy for sepsis.

The subcutaneous route can be used as it does not require particular techniques or surgical manipulation and therefore it may be an option as a route of delivery of the vector and could be clinically relevant. However, it remains unclear whether subcutaneous delivery of Adeno-β_2-AR might be effective in providing sustained and therapeutic levels of the transgene in the target organs. Furthermore, viral vectors have some negative characteristics, mainly that they can trigger inflammatory and immune responses with the possibility that adenovirus gene therapy may worsen the outcome of sepsis. With this in mind, we have undertaken the experiment [110] to explore whether the utilization of the subcutaneous injection technique could potentiate the β_2-AR signaling systems in the kidney and at the same time to test the safety of gene product. Furthermore, we have sought to evaluate its efficacy in preventing endotoxin-induced renal dysfunction.

The results from this experiment demonstrated that Adeno-β_2-AR (10^{10} t. v. p) delivery via the subcutaneous route was effective in providing sustained levels of the transgene in the target organ, of at least a doubling of the endogenous content for at least three weeks. Interestingly, a similar magnitude and pattern of changes in adrenoceptor content were also observed in the lung but to a lesser extent in the liver and heart. Importantly, it was evident from the physiological parameters, which is body weight, BP and plasma biochemistry that these were very comparable in the control and viral vector treated groups of rats and suggested that the vector had no untoward effect at least in the three week time frame. Moreover, the histological evaluation of the kidney, lung, liver, and heart showed that a 10^{10} t. v. p dose of Adeno-β_2-AR did not produce any evidence of cellular deterioration or toxicity using this adenoviral approach. It has been reported that adenoviral gene therapy induced a proinflammatory response in the lung and liver, characterized by increased TNF-α expression [111, 112] However, under the conditions of this study there was no elevation in TNF-α mRNA levels as a consequence of the Adeno-β_2-AR administration. Furthermore, this study showed that the plasma cytokine levels were not increased in the Adeno-β_2-AR treated rats. Together, these findings provide support for the view that Adeno-β_2-AR (10^{10} t. v. p) delivery via the subcutaneous route did not initiate any inflammatory responses at least over the three week period of observation. Nevertheless, the possibility remains that over a longer time frame integrating adenoviral vectors into the body might carry a greater risk of malignancy due to their ability to randomly integrate into the target genomes. An important outcome is that further basic study will be required to improve and further evaluate the technical aspects of the gene therapy using adenoviral vectors.

(4) Other gene therapies to sepsis

Some investigators have evaluated the effect of adenoviral vector gene transfer in animal models to overcome the consequences of sepsis. Alexander et al [113] demonstrated that adenoviral gene transfer of human bactericidal/permeability increasing protein (BPI) inhibited the effect of a non lethal dose of LPS on cytokine responses and improved the survival of mice subject to lethal septic shock. On the basis of these results, they suggested that human BPI gene transfer had the potential of being used as a therapeutic agent for septic conditions. In addition, Minter et al [114] reported that adenoviral expression of the anti-inflammatory cytokine IL-10 could be successfully used in the treatment of two acute inflammatory disease situations, for example, necrotizing pancreatitis and multisystem organ failure. However, whether these in vivo gene therapies prevented the progression of organ dysfunction associated with endotoxemia remains unclear. It was of concern that although administration of these genes effectively supported organ functions, these gene therapies were not able to survive all of the endotoxemic animals. Therefore, the gene therapy and adjuvant supportive cares therapy and early administration of empirical antibiotic therapy may be also required to improve the survival of the patients with sepsis [115].

CONCLUSION

Sepsis caused by bacteria and toxin is a common cause of ARF resulting in a high mortality rate in children. Cytokine production and release, HSP expression, nitric oxide synthesis activity, coagulation factors or factors of the innate immune system-like defenses involved in inflammation, contribute to a wide range of clinical manifestations of an inflammatory disease. Interestingly, functional β_2-AR activation is also involved in SIRS associated with endotoxemia and HUS and contributes to the treatment of some inflammatory diseases, including sepsis. Importantly, it was reported that cAMP-PKA activation is a central component in the protection against endotoxin-induced ARF. The β_2-AR activation could potentially be an important genetic factor pre-determining the degree of pathobiology of endotoxin-induced ARF and Stx-induced HUS. Importantly, constitutive β_2-AR activation after the Adeno-β_2-AR gene delivery was able to protect renal function through several mechanisms, including the cAMP-PKA pathway. The model presented herein is of *in vivo* gene transfer of Adeno-β_2-AR into the kidney, which has been demonstrated to be an efficient and reproducible global delivery of transgene to the renal glomeruli and tubular epithelial cells of the rat (Figure 6). In this model, we present novel findings indicating that the delivery of Adeno-β_2-AR gene is a potential novel therapeutic strategy for treatment of ARF associated with sepsis. Together, these findings suggest that functional β_2-AR activation may be a potential prophylactic/therapeutic approach in patients at high risk of developing ARF or patients who suffer sepsis but have not yet developed renal failure.

(A)   (B)

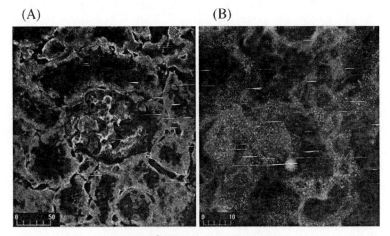

adeno-β2AR in the glomeruli

Figure 6. Immunohistochemical detection of β_2-AR expressed in the right kidney 4 wk after intraparenchymal injection (10^9 t. v. p.) of Adeno-β_2-AR–treated rats. β_2-AR was not only expressed in renal tubules (A: Scale bars: 50 μm) but also in glomeruli (B: Scale bars: 10 μm). White signals in the cells indicate β_2-AR expression.

ACKNOWLEDGEMENTS

I am very grateful for support from a Grant-in-Aid for Scientific Research from the Ministry of Education, Sports, Science and Technology, Japan (17590845) and Kawano Masanori Memorial Foundation for Promotion of Pediatrics. I thank Prof. E.J.Johns. Department of Physiology, University of Cork, Ireland, for critical review of the manuscript and suggestions and Mrs. Kumiko Kurosaki for technical support.

REFERENCES

[1]   Christenson, J. T., Sigurdsson, G. H., Mousawi, M. & Owunwanne, A. (1987). Use of indium-111 oscine to study the effects of terbutaline on pulmonary and hepatic plateletsequestration in endotoxin shock. Am. J. Physiol. Imaging, 2, 186-191.

[2]   Gluser, M. P., Zanetti, G., Baumgartner, J. D. & Cohen, J. (1991). Septic shock: pathogenesis. *Lancet, 338,* 732-736.

[3]   Nakamura, A., Johns, E. J., Imaizumi, A., Yanagawa, Y. & Kohsaka, T. (2001). Activation of β-adrenoceptor prevents shiga toxin-induced tumour necrosis factor production. *J. Am. Soc. Nephrol, 12,* 2288-2299.

[4]   Nakamura, A., Imaizumi, A., Yanagawa, Y., Kohsaka, T. & Johns, E. J. (2004). β_2-Adrenoceptor activation attenuates endotoxin-induced acute renal failure. *J. Am. Soc. Nephrol, 15,* 316–325.

[5]   Collins, F. S. (1999). Shattuck lecture: medical and societal consequences of the Human Genome Project. *N. Engl. J. Med, 341,* 28-37.

[6]   Liano, F., Junco, E., Madero, R., Pascual, J. & Verde, E. (1998). The spectrum of acute renal failure in the intensive care unit compared with that seen in other settings. The Madrid Acute renal Failure Study Group. *Kidney Int., 66,* S16-S24.

[7]   Schor, N. (2002). Acute renal failure and the sepsis syndrome. *Kidney Int., 61,* 764-776.

[8]   Kikeri, D., Pennel, J. P., Hwang, K. H., Jakob, J. I., Richman, A. V. & Bourgigne, J. J. (1986). Endotoxemic acute renal failure in awake rats. *Am. J. Physiol, 250,* F1098-F1106.

[9]   Zager, R. A. (1986). Escherichia coli endotoxin injections potentiate experimental ischemic renal injury. *Am. J. Physiol, 251,* F988-F994.

[10]   Kaplan, S. L. (1998). Bacteremia and septic shock in *Textbook of Pediatric Infectious Diseases, (4).* Edited by Feigin, R. D. & Cherry, J. D. Philadelphia, WB Saunders, 807-820.

[11]   Wiecek, A., Zeier, M. & Ritz, E. (1994). Role of infection in the genesis of acute renal failure. *Nephrol. Dial. Transplant, 4,* 40-44.

[12]   Boim, M. A., dos Santos, O. F., Barros, E. J. & Schor, N. (1997). Glomerular hemodynamics in acute renal failure. *Ren. Fail, 19,* 209-212.

[13]   Camussi, G., Ronco, C., Montrucchio, G. & Piccoli, G. (1998). Role of soluble mediators in sepsis and renal failure. *Kidney Int., 53,* S66 , S38–S42.

[14]   Casey, L. C. B. R. & Bone, R. C. (1993). Plasma cytokine and endotoxin levels correlate with survival in patients with the sepsis syndrome. *Ann. Intern. Med, 119,* 771–778.

[15] Pinsky, M. R. V. J., Deviere, J., Alegre, M., Kahn, R. J. & Dupont, E. (1993) Serum cytokine levels in human septic shock. Relation to multiple-system organ failure and mortality. *Chest, 103*, 565–575.

[16] Bone, R. C. & Newton, I. (1996). SEPSIS, SIRS, and CARS. *Crit. Care. Med., 24* , 1125–1128.

[17] Jaber, B. L. & Pereira, B. J. G. (1996). Inflammatory mediators in sepsis: rationale for extracorporeal therapies. *Am. J. Kidney Dis., 28* , S35–S49.

[18] Thijs, A. & Thijs, L. G. (1998). Pathogenesis of renal failure in sepsis. *Kidney Int., 66*, S34–S37.

[19] Uddman, E., Moller, S., Adner, M. & Edvinsson, L. (1999). Cytokines induce increased endothelin ET(B) receptor-mediated contraction. *Eur. J. Pharmacol, 376*, 223–232.

[20] Tschaikowsky, K., Sagner, S., Lehnert, N., Kaul, M. & Ritter, J. (2000). Endothelin in septic patients: effects on cardiovascular and renal function and its relationship to proinflammatory cytokines. *Crit. Care. Med, 28*, 1854–1860.

[21] Flo, T. H., Halaas, O., Torp, S., Ryan, L., Lien, E., Dybdahl, B., Sundan, A. & Espevik, T. (2001). Differential expression of Toll-like receptor 2 in human cells. *J. Leukoc. Biol, 69*, 474-481.

[22] Cunningham, P. N., Dyanov, H. M., Park, P., Wang, J., Newell, K. A. & Quigg, R. J. (2002). Acute renal failure in endotoxemia is caused by TNF acting directly on TNF receptor-1 in kidney. *J. Immun, 168*, 5817-5823.

[23] Bonventre, J. V. & Weinberg, J. M. (2003). Recent advances in the pathophysiology of ischemic acute renal failure. *J. Am. Soc. Nephrol, 14*, 2199-210.

[24] Linas, S. L., Whittenburg, D., Parsons, P. E. & Repine, J. E. (1992). Mild renal ischemia activates primed neutrophils to cause acute renal failure. *Kidney Int, 42*, 610-616.

[25] Bernard, G. R., Vincent, J. L. & Laterre, P. F. (2001). Efficacy and safety of recombinant human activated protein C for severe sepsis. *N. Engl. J. Med, 344*, 699-709.

[26] Jaber, B. L., Madhumathi, R., Daqing, G., Vaidyanathapuram, S., Perianayagam, M. C., Freeman, R. B. & Pereira, B. J. (2004). Cytokine gene promoter polymorphisms and mortality in acute renal failure. *Cytokine, 25*, 212-219.

[27] Fekete, A., Treszl, A., Toth-Heyn, P., Vannay, A., Tordai, A., Tulassay, T. & Vasarhelyi, B. (2003). Association between heat shock protein 72 gene polymorphism and acute renal failure in premature neonates. *Pediatr. Res, 54*, 452-455.

[28] Vicencio, A., Bidmon, B., Ryu, J., Reidy, K., Thulin, G., Mann, A., Gaudio, K. M., Kashgarian, M. & Siegel, N. J. (2003). Developmental expression of HSP-72 and ischemic tolerance of the immature kidney. *Pediatr. Nephrol, 18*, 85–91.

[29] Vasarhelyi, B., Toth-Heyn, P., Treszl, A. & Tulassay, T. (2005). Genetic polymorphisms and risk for acute renal failure in preterm neonates. *Pediatr. Nephrol., 20*, 132-135.

[30] Stuber, F., Petersen, M., Bokelmann, F. & Schade, U. (1996). A genomic polymorphism within the tumor necrosis factor locus influences plasma tumor necrosis factor-β concentrations and outcome of patients with severe sepsis. *Crit. Care. Med, 24*, 381-384.

[31] Fang, X. M., Schroder, S., Hoeft, A. & Stuber, F. (1999). Comparison of two polymorphisms of the interleukin-1 gene family: interleukin-1 receptor antagonist

polymorphism contributes to susceptibility to severe sepsis. *Crit. Care. Med, 27*, 1330-1334.

[32] Treszl, A., Toth-Heyn, P., Kocsis, I., Nobilis, A., Schuler, A., Tulassay, T. & Vasarhelyi, B. (2002). Interleukin genetic variants and the risk of renal failure in infants with infection. *Pediatr. Nephrol, 17*, 713-717.

[33] Lowe, P. R., Galley, H. F., Abdel-Fattah, A. & Webster, N. R. (2003). Influence of interleukin-10 polymorphisms on interleukin-10 expression and survival in critically ill patients. *Crit. Care. Med, 31*, 34-38.

[34] Gibot, S., Cariou, A., Drouet, L., Rossignol, M. & Ripoll, L. (2002). Association between a genomic polymorphism within the CD14 locus and septic shock susceptibility and mortality rate. *Crit. Care Med, 30*, 969-973.

[35] Waterer, G. W., ElBahlawan, L., Quasney, M. W., Zhang, Q., Kessler, L. A. & Wunderink, R. G. (2003). Heat shock protein 70-2+1267 AA homozygotes have an increased risk of septic shock in adults with community-acquired pneumonia. *Crit. Care. Med, 31*, 1367-1372.

[36] Child, N. J., Yang, I. A., Pulletz, M. C., de Courcy-Golder, K., Andrews, A. L., Pappachan, V. J. & Holloway, J. W. (2003). Polymorphisms in Toll-like receptor 4 and the systemic inflammatory response syndrome. *Biochem. Soc. Trans, 31*, 652-3.

[37] Ader, R., Cohen, N. & Felten, D. (1995). Psychoneuroimmunology: interactions between the nervous system and the immune system. *Lancet, 345*, 99–103.

[38] Bergquist, J., Tarkowski, A., Ekman, R. & Ewing, A. (1994). Discovery of endogenous catecholamines in lymphocytes and evidence for catecholamine regulation of lymphocyte function via an autocrine loop. *Proc. Natl. Acad. Sci. U. S. A., 91*, 12912–12916.

[39] Josefsson, E., Bergquist, J., Ekman, R. & Tarkowski, A. (1996). Catecholamines are synthesized by mouse lymphocytes and regulate function of these cells by induction of apoptosis. *Immunology, 88*, 140–146.

[40] Sanders, V. M., Baker, R. A., Ramer-Quinn, D. S., Kasprowicz, D. J., Fuchs, B. A. & Street, N. E. (1997). Differential expression of the β_2-adrenergic receptor by Th1 and Th2 clones: implications for cytokine production and B cell help. *J. Immunol, 158*, 4200–4210.

[41] Gaballa, M. A., Peppel, K., Lefkowitz, R. J., Aguirre, M., Dolber, P. C., Pennock, G. D., Koch, W. J. & Goldman, S. (1998). Enhanced vasorelaxation by overexpression of β_2-adrenergic receptors in large arteries. *J. Mol Cell Cardiol, 30*, 1037–1045.

[42] Chruscinski, A. J., Rohrer, D. K., Schauble, E., Desai, K. H., Bernstein, D. & Kobilka, B. K. (1999). Targeted disruption of the β_2 adrenergic receptor gene. *J. Biol. Chem., 274*, 16694–16700.

[43] Iaccarino, G., Cipolletta, E., Fiorillo, A., Annecchiarico, M., Ciccarelli, M., Cimini, V., Koch, W. J. & Trimarco, B. (2002). β_2-adrenergic receptor gene delivery to the endothelium corrects impaired adrenergic vasorelaxation in hypertension. *Circulation, 106*, 349-355.

[44] Nakamura, A., Niimi, R. & Yanagawa, Y. (2007). Renal effects of β_2-adrenoceptor agonist and clinical analysis in children. *Pediatr Res, 61*, 129-133.

[45] Nakamura, A., Imaizumi, A., Kohsaka, T., Yanagawa, Y. & Johns, E. J. (2000). β_2-adrenoceptor agonist suppresses tumour necrosis factor production in rat mesangial cells. *Cytokine, 12*, 491-494.

[46] Liao, J., Keiser, J. A., Scales, W. E., Kunkel, S. L. & Kluger, M. J. (1995). Role of epinephrine in TNF and IL-6 production from isolated perfused rat liver. *Am. J. Physiol, 268*, R896-R901.

[47] Severn, A., Rapson, N. T., Hunter, C. A. & Liew, F. Y. (1992). Regulation of tumor necrosis factor production by adrenaline and β-adrenergic agonists. *J. Immunol, 148*, 3441-3445.

[48] Hetier, P., Ayala, J., Bousseau, A. & Prochiantz, A. (1991). Modulation of interleukin-1 and tumor necrosis factor expression by β-adrenergic agonists in mouse ameboid microgial cells. *Exp. Brain Res, 86*, 407-413.

[49] Bernardin, G., Strosberg, A. D., Bernard, A., Mattei, M. & Marullo, S. (1998). Beta-adrenergic receptor-dependent and -independent stimulation of adenylate cyclase is impaired during severe sepsis in humans. *Intensive Care Med, 24*, 1315-1322

[50] Schmidt, W., Hacker, A., Gebhard, M. M., Martin, E. & Schmidt, H. (1998). Dopexamine attenuates endotoxin-induced microcirculatory changes in rat mesentery: role of β_2 adrenoceptors. *Crit. Care. Med, 26*, 1639-1645.

[51] Tighe, D., Moss, R. & Bennett, D. (1996). Cell surface adrenergic receptor stimulation modifies the endothelial response to SIRS. Systemic Inflammatory Response Syndrome. *New Horiz, 4*, 426-442.

[52] Tighe, D., Moss, R. & Bennett, D. (1998). Porcine hepatic response to sepsis and its amplification by an adrenergic receptor alpha1 agonist and a β_2 antagonist. *Clin. Sci (Lond).*, *95*, 467-478.

[53] Sigurdsson, G. H., Christenson, J. T., al-Mousawi, M. & Owunwanne, A. (1989). Use of indium-111 oxine to study pulmonary and hepatic leukocyte sequestration in endotoxin shock and effects of the β_2 receptor agonist terbutaline. *Am. J. Physiol Imaging, 4*, 136-142.

[54] Nakamura, A. & Yanagawa, Y. (2008). Pharmacogenomics and sepsis-induced renal failure: Effects of β_2-adrenoceptor function on the course of sepsis. *Current Pharmacogenomics and Personalized Medicine, 6*, 98-107.

[55] Nakamura, A., Imaizumi, A., Yanagawa, Y., Niimi, R. & Kohsaka, T. (2003). Suppression of tumor necrosis factor-alpha by β_2-adrenoceptor activation: role of mitogen-activated protein kinases in renal mesangial cells. *Inflammation Res., 52*, 26-31.

[56] Nakamura, A., Johns, E. J., Imaizumi, A., Yanagawa, Y. & Kohsaka, T. (1999). Effect of β_2-adrenoceptor activation and angiotensin II on tumour necrosis factor and interleukin-6 genes transcription in the rat renal resident macrophage cells. *Cytokine, 11*, 759–65.

[57] Weiss, M., Schneider, E. M., Tarnow, J. Mettler, S. Krone, M. Teschemacher, A, & Lemoine H. (1996). Is inhibition of oxygen radical production of neutrophils by sympathomimetics mediated via β_2 adrenoceptors? *J. Pharmacol Exp. Ther, 278*, 1105-1113.

[58] Svensjo, E., Persson, C. G. & Rutili, G. (1977). Inhibition of bradykinin-induced macromolecular leakage from postcapillary venules by a β_2-AR stimulant, terbutaline. *Acta. Physiol. Scand, 101*, 504-506.

[59] Makhlouf, K., Comabella, M., Imitola, J., Weiner, H. L. & Khoury, S. J. (2001). Oral salbutamol decreases IL-12 in patients with secondary progressive multiple sclerosis. *J. Neuroimmunol, 117*, 156–165.

[60] Malfait, A. M., Malik, A. S., Marinova-Mutafchieva, L., Butler, D. M., Maini, R. N. & Feldmann, M. (1999). The β_2-adrenergic agonist salbutamol is a potent suppressor of established collagen-induced arthritis: mechanisms of action. *J. Immunol, 162*, 6278–6283.

[61] Tiegs, G., Bang, R. & Neuhuber, W. L. (1999). Requirement of peptidergic sensory innervation for disease activity in murine models of immune hepatitis and protection by β-adrenergic stimulation. *J. Neuroimmunol, 96*, 131–143.

[62] Van der Poll, T., Coyle, S. M., Barbosa, K., Braxton, C. C. & Lowry, S. F. (1996). Epinephrine inhibits tumor necrosis factor-β and potentiates interleukin-10 production during human endotoxemia. *J. Clin. Invest, 97*, 713-719.

[63] Van der Pouw-Kraan, T. C. T. M., Boeije, L. C. M., Smeenk, R. J. T., Wijdenes, J. & Aarden, L. A. (1995). Prostaglandin-E_2 is a potent inhibitor of human interleukin 12 production. *J. Exp. Med, 181*, 775-779.

[64] Strassmann, G., Patil-Koota, V., Finkelman, F., Fong, M. & Kambayashi, T. (1994). Evidence for the involvement of interleukin 10 in the differential deactivation of murine peritoneal macrophages by prostaglandin E_2. *J. Exp. Med., 180*, 2365-2370.

[65] Panina-Bordignon, P. J., Mazzeo, D., Di Lucia, P. D'Ambrosio, D. Lang, R. Fabbri, L. Self, C. & Sinigaglia, F. (1997). β_2-agonists prevent Th1 development by selective inhibition of interleukin 12. *J. Clin. Invest, 100*, 1513–1519.

[66] Koepke, J. P. & Dibona, G. F. (1986). Central adrenergic receptor control of renal function in conscious hypertensive rats. *Hypertension, 8*, 133–141.

[67] Shimkets, R. A., Warnock, D. G., Bositis, C. M., Nelson-Williams, C., Hansson, J. H., Schambelan, M. Gill, Jr. Ulick, S. Milora, R. V. & Findling, J. W. (1994). Liddle's syndrome: heritable human hypertension caused by mutations in the β subunit of the epithelial sodium channel. *Cell, 79*, 407–414.

[68] DiBona, G. F. & Kopp, U. C. (1997). Neural control of renal function. *Physiol. Rev., 77*, 75–197.

[69] Boivin, V., Jahns, R., Gambaryan, S., Ness, W., Boege, F. & Lohse, M. J. (2001). Immunofluorescent imaging of β_1- and β_2-adrenergic receptors in rat kidney. *Kidney Int., 59*, 515-531.

[70] Pradervand, S., Barker, P. M., Wang, Q. & Ernst, S. A. (1999). Beermann F., Grubb B. R., Burnier M., Schmidt A., Bindels R. J., Gatzy J. T., Rossier B. C., Hummler E. Salt restriction induces pseudohypoaldosteronism type 1 in mice expressing low levels of the β-subunit of the amiloride-sensitive epithelial sodium channel. *Proc. Natl. Acad. Sci. U. S. A., 96*, 1732–1737.

[71] Snyder, P. M. (2000). Liddle's syndrome mutations disrupt cAMP-mediated translocation of the epithelial Na^+ channel to the cell surface. *J. Clin. Invest, 105*, 45–53.

[72] Wallace, D. P., Reif, G., Hedge, A. M., Thrasher, J. B. & Pietrow, P. (2004). Adrenergic regulation of salt and fluid secretion in human medullary collecting duct cells. *Am. J. Physiol. Renal Physiol, 287,* F639–F648.

[73] Tago, K. & Schuster, V. L. & Stokes, J. B. (1986). Regulation of chloride self exchange by cAMP in cortical collecting tubule. *Am. J. Physiol, 251,* F40-48.

[74] Singh, H. & Linas, S. (1997). Role of protein kinase C in β_2-adrenoceptor function in cultured rat proximal tubular epithelial cells. *Am. J. Physiol, 273,* F193-F199.

[75] Hashimoto, K., Shintani, S., Yamashita, S., Tei, S., Takai, M., Tsutsui, M., Kawamura, K., Ohkawa, T., Hiyama, T. & Yabuuchi, Y. (1979). Pharmacological properties of procaterol, a newly synthetized, specific β_2-adrenoceptor stimulant. Part II. Effects on the peripheral organs (author's transl). *Nippon Yakurigaku Zasshi, 75,* 333-364. (Japanese).

[76] Main, I. W., Nikolic-paterson, D. J. & Atkins, R. C. (1992). T cells and macrophages and their role in renal injury. *Semin Nephrol, 12,* 395-407.

[77] Klahr, S. (1993). Interstitial macrophages. *Semin Nephrol, 13,* 388-395.

[78] Fougueray, B., Philipp, C., Herbelin, A. & Perez, J., Ardaillov, R. & Baud, L. (1993). Cytokine formation within rat glomeruli during experimental endotoxaemia. *J. Am. Soc. Nephrol, 3,* 1783-1791.

[79] Kayama, E., Yoshida, T., Kodama, Y., Matsui, T., Matheson, J. M. & Luster, M. I. (1997). Proinflammatory cytokines and interleukin-6 in the renal response to bacterial endotoxin. *Cytokine, 9,* 688-695.

[80] Nakamura. A., Johns, E. J., Imaizumi, A., Yanagawa, Y. & Kohsaka, T. (1999). Modulation of interleukin-6 by β_2-adrenoceptor in endotoxin-stimulated renal macrophage. *Kidney Int., 56,* 839-849.

[81] Hirano, T. & Kishimoto, T. (1990). Interleukin-6. In *Handbook of Experimental Pharmacology, (95)* edited by Sporn MB, Roberts AB, Berlin, Springer-Verlag, 633-665.

[82] Maimone, D. C., Cioni, C., Rosa, S., Machia, G., Aloisi, F. & Annunziata, P. (1993). Norepinephrine and vasoactive intestinal peptide induce interleukin-6 secretion by astrocytes. *J. Neuroimmunol, 47,* 73-81.

[83] Zhang, Y., Lin, Jian-Xin. J. & Vilcek, J. (1988). Synthesis of interleukin-6 in human fibroblasts is triggered by increase in intracellular cyclic AMP. *J. Biol. Chem., 263,* 6177-6182.

[84] Straub, R. H., Hermann, M., Frauenholz, T., Berkmiller, G., Lang, B., Scholmerich, J and Falk, W. (1996). Neuroimmune control of interleukin-6 secretion in the murine spleen. *J. Neuroimmunol, 71,* 37-43

[85] Nakamura, A., Johns, E. J., Imaizumi, A., Abe, T. & Kohsaka, T. (1998). Regulation of tumour necrosis factor and interleukin-6 gene transcription by beta2-adrenoceptor in the rat astrocytes. *J. Neuroimmunol, 88,* 144-153.

[86] Kaplan, B. S., Meyers, K. E. & Schulman, S. L. (1998). The pathogeneis and treatment of hemolytic uremic syndrome. *J. Am. Soc. Nephrol, 8,* 1126-1133.

[87] Fong, J. S., De Chadarevian, J. P. & Kaplan, B. S. (1982). Hemolytic Uremic Syndrome. Current concepts and management. *Pediatr. Clin. N. Am., 29,* pp. 835–856.

[88] Van De Kar, N. C., Monnens, L. A., Karmali, M. A. & Van Hinsbergh, V. W. (1992). Tumour necrosis factor and interleukin-1 induce expression of the verocytotoxin

receptor globotriaosylceramide on human vascular endothelial cells: Implications for the pathogenesis of the hemolytic uremic syndrome. *Blood, 80,* 2755-2764.

[89] Lingwood, C. A. (1994). Verotoxin-binding in human renal sections. *Nephron, 66,* 21 – 28.

[90] Kiyokawa, N., Taguchi, T., Mori, T., Uchida, H., Sato, N., Takeda, T. & Fujimoto, J. (1998). Induction of apoptosis in normal human renal tubular epithelial cells by Escherichia coli shiga toxin 1 and 2. *J. Infect Dis., 178,* 178-184.

[91] Hughes, A. K., Stricklett, P. K. & Kohan, D. E. (1998). Cytotoxic effect of shiga toxin-1 on human proximal tubule cells. *Kidney Int., 54,* 426-437.

[92] Zhu, Y., Prehn, J. H. M., Culmsee, C. & Krieglstein, J. (1999). The β₂-adrenoceptor agonist clenbuterol modulates Bcl-2, Bcl-xl and Bax protein expression following transient forebrain ischemia. *Neuroscience, 90,* 1255-1263.

[93] Nakamura, A., Imaizumi, A., Yanagawa, Y., Niimi, R., Kohsaka, T. & Johns, E. J. (2003). β₂-adrenoceptor activation inhibits Shiga toxin2-induced apoptosis of renal tubular epithelial cells. *Biochem Pharmacol, 66,* 343-53.

[94] Beutler, B. (2000). TRL4: central component of the sole mammalian LPS sensor. *Curr Opin Immunol, 12,* 20-6.

[95] Poltorak, A., He, X., Smirnova, I., Liu, M. Y., Van Huffel, C., Du, X. Birdwell, D. Alejos, E. Silva, M. Galanos, C. Freudenberg, M. Ricciardi-Castagnoli, P. Layton, B. & Beutler, B. (1998). Defective LPS signaling in C3H/HeJ and C57BL/10ScCr mice: mutations in Tlr4 gene. *Science, 282,* 2085-8.

[96] Chen, G., Li, J., Ochani, M., Rendon-Mitchell, B., Qiang, X., Susarla, S., Ulloa, L.,Yang, H., Fan, S., Goyert, S. M., Wang, P., Tracey, K. J., Sama, A. E., and Wang, H. (2004). Bacterial endotoxin stimulates macrophages to release HMGB1 partly through CD14- and TNF-dependent mechanisms. *J. Leukoc Biol, 76,* 994-1001.

[97] Cunningham, P. N., Wang, Y., Guo, R., He, G. & Quigg, R. J. (2004). Role of Toll-like receptor 4 in endotoxin-induced acute renal failure. *J. Immunol, 172,* 2629-35.

[98] Nakamura, A., Niimi, R. & Yanagawa, Y. (2009). Renal β₂-adrenoceptor modulates the lipopolysaccharide transport system in sepsis-induced acute renal failure. *Inflammation, 32,*12-19.

[99] Nakamura, A., Johns, E. J., Imaizumi, A., Yanagawa, Y. & Kohsaka, T. (1997). β₂-adrenoceptor activation and angiotensin II regulate tumour necrosis factor and interleukin-6 genes transcription in the rat renal resident macrophage and mesangial cells. *J. Am. Soc. Nephrol, 8,* 479A (abstract)

[100] Nakamura, A., Johns, E. J., Imaizumi, A., Yanagawa, Y. & Kohsaka, T. (2000). β₂-adrenoceptor agonist suppresses renal tumour necrosis factor and enhances interleukin-6 gene expression induced by endotoxin. *Nephrol Dial Transplant., 15,* 1928-1934.

[101] Richardson, S. E., Karmali, M. A., Becker, L. E. & Smith, C. R. (1988). The histopathology of the hemolytic uremic syndrome associated with verocytotoxin-producing Escherichia coli infection. *Human Pathol, 19 ,* 1102-1108.

[102] Inward, C., Howie, A., Fitspatrick, M., Rafaat, F., Milford, D. & Taylor, C. M. (1997). Renal histopathology in fetal cases of diarrhea-associated hemolytic uremic syndrome. British Association of Paediatric Nephrology. *Pediatr Nephrol, 11,* 556 –559.

[103] Taguchi, T., Uchida, H., Kiyokawa, N., Mori, T., Sato, N., Horie, H., Takeda, T. & Fujimoto, J. (1998). Verotoxins induce apoptosis in human renal tubular epithelium derived cells. *Kidney Int .*, *53,*1681 –1688.

[104] Emilien, G. & Maloteaux, J. M. (1998). Current therapeutic uses and potential of beta-adrenoceptor agonists and antagonists. *Eur J. Clin. Pharmacol, 53,* 389–404.

[105] Maurice, L. P., Hata, J. A., Shah, A. S., White, D. C., McDonald, P. H., Dolber, P. C., Wilson, K. H., Lefkowitz, R. J., Glower, D. D. & Koch, W. J. (1999). Enhancement of cardiac function after adenoviral-mediated in vivo intracoronary $_2$-adrenergic receptor gene delivery. *J. Clin. Invest ,104,* 21–29.

[106] Begany, D. P., Carcillo, J. A., Herzer, W. A., Mi, Z. & Jackson, E. K. (1996). Inhibition of type IV phosphodiesterase by Ro 20-1724 attenuates endotoxin-induced acute renal failure. *J. Pharmacol Exp. Ther., 278,* 37-41.

[107] Guan, Z., Miller, S. B. & Greenwald, J. E. (1995). Zaprinast accelerates recovery from established acute renal failure in the rat. *Kidney Int., 47,* 1569–1575.

[108] Huard, J., Lochmuller, H., Acsadi, G., Jani, A., Massie, B. & Karpati, G. (1995). The route of administration is a major determinant of the transduction efficiency of rat tissues by adenoviral recombinants. *Gene Ther., 2,* 107–115

[109] Chuah, M. K., Collen, D. & Vanden Driessche, T. (2003). Biosafety of adenoviral vectors. Curr. *Gene Ther., 3,* 527–543

[110] Nakamura, A., Imaizumi, A., Yanagawa, Y., Niimi, R., Kohsaka, T. & Johns, E. J. (2005). Adenoviral delivery of the beta$_2$-adrenoceptor gene in sepsis. *Clin. Science, 109,* 503-511.

[111] Elkon, K. B., Liu, C. C., Gall, J. G. Trevejo, J., Marino, M. W., Abrahamsen, K. A., Song, X., Zhou, J. L., Old, L. J., Crystal, R. G., and Falck-Pedersen, E. (1997) . TNF-α plays a central role in immune-mediated clearance of adenoviral vectors. *Proc. Natl. Acad. Sci. U. S. A., 94,* 9814–9819 .

[112] Zhang, H. G., Zhou, T., Yang, C., Edwards, P. K., Curiel, D. T. & Mountz, J. D. (1998). Inhibition of TNF-α decreases inflammation and prolongs adenovirus gene expression in lung and liver. Hum. *Gene Ther., 9,* 1875–1884.

[113] Alexander, S., Bramson, J., Foley, R. & Xing, Z. (2004). Protection from endotoxemia by adenoviral-mediated gene transfer of human bactericidal/permeability-increasing protein. *Blood, 103,* 93–99.

[114] Minter, R. M., Ferry, M. A., Murday, M. E. Tannahill, C. L., Bahjat, F. R., Oberholzer, C., Oberholzer, A., LaFace, D., Hutchins, B., Wen, S., Shinoda, J., Copeland, E. M. 3rd, and Moldawer, L. L. (2001). Adenoviral delivery of human and viral IL-10 in murine sepsis. *J. Immunol., 167,* 1053–1059.

[115] Sparrow, A. & Willis, F. (2004). Management of septic shock in childhood. Emerg. Med. *Australasia, 16,* 125–134.

In: Sepsis: Symptoms, Diagnosis and Treatment ISBN: 978-1-60876-609-3
Editor: Joseph R. Brown, pp. 55-73 © 2010 Nova Science Publishers, Inc.

Chapter 3

WHAT'S IN THE PIPELINE
FOR THE TREATMENT OF SEPSIS?

Chan-Ho Lee and Sun-Mee Lee[*]

College of Pharmacy, Sungkyunkwan University, Suwon 440-746, Korea

ABSTRACT

Sepsis is a multifactorial disease for which the total number of cases is expected to reach one million in the United States by the year 2010. With the development of novel invasive surgical procedures, the number of sepsis cases has doubled in the past 20 years. Despite numerous randomized clinical trials involving tens of thousands of subjects, the effort to resolve the most challenging problem in intensive care remains elusive due to the complexity and rapid progression of the disease. Xigris®, the first FDA-approved drug for improving survival in patients with high-risk severe sepsis, failed to meet its high expectations due to its contraindications and its narrow label. There are also many examples of how recent research has led us astray. However, after a lengthy period of indecisive definitions of the disease, the healthcare industry is now addressing the major task of overcoming the unacceptable mortality caused by sepsis. This review provides an overview of medications that have not yet been approved for the treatment of patients with sepsis but have shown promise in clinical trials. These include drugs that target immunomodulation, the coagulation pathway, cell signaling, endotoxin, and specific mediators of sepsis. As the understanding of the disease has improved and the research into the development of therapeutic candidates has advanced, the expectations for a successful sepsis drug is now higher than ever. However, this will necessitate the development of an advanced diagnostic to specifically determine the condition of sepsis patients. The hope of providing relief to patients should encourage the healthcare industry to achieve these goals.

---

[*] Corresponding author: Tel.: +82 31 290 7712; fax: +82 31 292 8800. E-mail address: sunmee@skku.edu (S.-M. Lee).

1. INTRODUCTION

Sepsis accounts for almost 210,000 deaths and an estimated expenditure of $16 billion annually in the United States alone. Despite more than 70 multicenter clinical trials and a five-fold increase in basic research over the past two decades, only activated protein C (drotrecogin alfa) has received approval from the United States Food and Drug Administration for the treatment of sepsis [1]. Due to the delay in the development of new treatments, available therapies for sepsis are still limited to several simple clinical interventions: initial resuscitation (first 6 h); broad-spectrum antibiotics; steroidal anti-inflammatory drugs; adjunctive therapy with an anti-coagulant agent; and insulin therapy for glucose control.

However, encouraging new data have recently been presented on new approaches for the management of patients with sepsis. Many of these approaches attempt to modulate or interrupt the sepsis cascade and address the cause of multiple organ dysfunction syndrome. Although many of these approaches (e.g., targeting immunomodulation, the coagulation pathway, cell signaling, endotoxin, and specific mediators of sepsis, etc.) are in the early phases of development, they provide new insight into the treatment of sepsis. Here, we review the emerging pharmacological treatments for sepsis and describe the current status of sepsis research.

2. BACKGROUND

Sepsis is the culmination of complex interactions between the infecting microorganism and the host immune, inflammatory, and coagulation responses. The rationale for the use of therapeutic targets in sepsis has arisen from concepts of pathogenesis.

2.1. Innate and Adaptive Immunity in Sepsis

Invasion and proliferation of microorganisms are initial steps in the pathological process in septic patients. When the pathogens cross the host's natural barrier, defense mechanisms including both innate and adaptive immune responses are activated in a sequential manner. Immune cells express pattern-recognition receptors (PRRs) on their surface, which recognize and interact with pathogen-associated molecular patterns (PAMPs) [2].

It should be noted that the initiation of the host response during sepsis involves various PRR families including toll-like receptors (TLRs). In fact, recent evidence shows the crucial role of TLRs in septic patients, especially TLR-2 and TLR-4 [3-5]. Other components of the cellular innate recognition system include scavenger receptors, the cell-surface protein MD-2, the triggering receptor expressed on myeloid cells (TREM-1), and the monocyte intracellular proteins NOD-1 and NOD-2 [2,6,7].

Microorganisms also stimulate specific humoral and cell-mediated adaptive immune responses that amplify innate immunity. B cells produce immunoglobulin, which is responsible for facilitating delivery of microorganisms to antigen presenting cells to natural killer cells. T cells, both type 1 helper T cells (Th1) and type 2 helper T cells (Th2), are involved in cytokine production. Generally, Th1 cells release pro-inflammatory cytokines such as TNF-α while Th2 cells secrete anti-inflammatory cytokines such as IL-4 and IL-10 [8].

2.2. Disturbance of the Coagulation Pathway

The altered coagulation homeostasis is important in sepsis and is typically accompanied by increased pro-coagulant factors and decreased anti-coagulant factors. During the systemic inflammatory response such as in sepsis, the bacterial component lipopolysaccaride (LPS) as well as inflammatory cytokines such as TNF-α and IL-1 up-regulate tissue factor (TF) release from endothelial cells, activating coagulation. Activated protein C, an endogenous plasma serine protease, exerts important antithrombotic activities by inactivating Factors Va and VIIIa, which limits thrombin generation and reduces its pro-coagulant and anti-fibrinolytic properties [9]. Unfortunately, sepsis lowers the levels of protein C and other anti-coagulant factors including protein S, antithrombin III, and tissue factor-pathway inhibitor. Clinical data shows frequent occurrence of disseminated intravascular coagulation (DIC) in septic patients [10]. There is little doubt that DIC leads to microvascular thrombosis throughout the body, impairing perfusion of critical organs.

2.3. Inflammatory Response in Early Sepsis and Anti-Inflammatory Cascade/Apoptosis in Late Sepsis

Following the initial host-microbial interaction, there is widespread activation of the innate immune response. Mononuclear cells play a key role, releasing pro-inflammatory cytokines IL-1, IL-6 and TNF-α. Thus, the early state of sepsis is characterized by increased inflammatory cytokines, a so-called "cytokine storm". However, sepsis is much more complex than initially thought. Indeed, as sepsis persists, the disease state shifts toward an anti-inflammatory immunosuppressive state.

Although many cytokines play a role in the early phase of sepsis, TNF-α appears to predominate in the initial phases. In addition to being the first cytokine released into circulation during the inflammatory response, when administered to humans, TNF-α also induces many of the pathogenic alterations associated with sepsis [11-13]. Once released, TNF-α stimulates the additional cytokines IL-6 and IL-8. TNF-α, in conjunction with other cytokines, up-regulates adhesion molecules (e.g., ICAM-1, ICAM-2, P-selectin, E-selectin) in neutrophils and endothelial cells. High-mobility group box 1 (HMGB1), a non-histone chromosomal protein, has recently been identified as a cytokine-like product of macrophages that is also known as a late mediator of sepsis [14]. HMGB1 has pro-inflammatory effects and triggers apoptotic tissue damage, and is also involved in the amplification of other cytokines through TLR signaling [15,16].

As previously mentioned, the initial hyper-inflammatory response in sepsis is quickly followed by the sustained anti-inflammatory/immunosuppressive state that has been termed 'immune paralysis'. In this late stage of sepsis, anti-inflammatory molecules IL-10, transforming growth factor, IL-13, soluble cytokine inhibitors IL-1ra, sIL-1ra, and sTNFR parallel the excessive production of pro-inflammatory cytokines. Substantial investigations have also defined the key role of apoptosis as one of the major mechanisms of the anti-inflammatory host response during sepsis [17,18].

2.4. Multiple Organ Dysfunction Syndrome and Sepsis

The aberrant signaling pathways in sepsis ultimately lead to tissue injury and multiple organ dysfunction syndrome. Organ failure often begins with respiratory failure, followed by intestinal, hepatic, renal, hematologic, and cardiac failure; the exact order may vary because of preexisting disease or the nature of the precipitating insult [19].

3. CURRENT MANAGEMENT OF SEPSIS

3.1. Volume Resuscitation

The "Surviving Sepsis Campaign: International guidelines for management of severe sepsis and septic shock: 2008" states that immediate resuscitation should be provided to patients with hypotension or elevated serum lactate levels (>4 mmol/l) [20]. Resuscitation goals are central venous pressure of 8-12 mmHg; mean arterial pressure greater than or equal to 65 mmHg; increased urine output ($\geq$0.5 ml/kg/h); and 70% central venous oxygen saturation.

Early aggressive therapy that optimizes cardiac preload, afterload, and contractility in patients with severe sepsis and septic shock improves the likelihood of survival [21]. Infusions of colloid or crystalloid, vasoactive agents, and transfusions of red cells to increase oxygen delivery can also be helpful. Mortality was 30.5% in the group receiving early goal-directed treatment compared with 46.5% in the control group (P=0.009). Thus, early therapeutic intervention to restore the balance between oxygen delivery and oxygen demand improves survival among patients presenting with severe sepsis.

3.2. Antibiotics

With the identification of infection, broad-spectrum antibiotics are immediately administered to patients [20]. Early adequate antibiotic treatment reduced mortality in bacteremic patients but this was not as obvious in a study of critically ill patients [22]. By multivariate analysis, the risk of in-hospital mortality was eight times greater in cases of inadequate antimicrobial therapy within the first 24 h. A study by MacArthur *et al.* [23] showed a 33% mortality rate in patients with suspected sepsis who received adequate antibiotics therapy compared with a 43% mortality in patients who did not. However, administration of antibiotics may also trigger the release of bacterial products, for example, endotoxin, that may further stimulate innate immune cells to release inflammatory cytokines.

3.3. Steroidal Anti-Inflammatory Drugs

Although high-dose steroid may worsen outcomes by increasing secondary infections [24], low-dose steroid therapy (50 mg hydrocortisone every 6 h, 50 µg oral fludrocortisones for 7 days) was beneficial in septic patients with adrenal insufficiency, despite elevated levels of circulating cortisol [25]. Combination therapy was beneficial even in patients with elevated base-line plasma cortisol levels if their serum cortisol level did not increase by more than 9 µg/dl when stimulated by adrenocorticotropic hormone. However, high-dose corticosteroid therapy should generally be avoided in treating patients with sepsis, as patients who did not have adrenal insufficiency and who received corticosteroids had a slight trend toward increased mortality [26].

3.4. Adjunctive Therapy with an Anti-Coagulant Agent; Activated Protein C

Activated protein C inactivates factors Va and VIIIa, thereby preventing the generation of thrombin, a major regulator of hemostasis [27]. Inhibition of thrombin generation by activated protein C decreases inflammation by inhibiting platelet activation, neutrophil recruitment, and mast-cell degranulation. Activated protein C has direct anti-inflammatory properties, including blocking of cytokine production by monocytes and blocking of cell adhesion.

Recombinant human activated protein C (drotrecogin alfa) is the first agent that has proved effective in the treatment of sepsis [28]. In patients with sepsis, the administration of activated protein C reduced 28-day mortality (from 30.8% in the placebo group to 24.7% in the drotrecogin alfa group); however, this was accompanied by a 1.5% increase in hemorrhagic complication risk. This has led to the approval of Xigris® (drotrecogin alfa) only for patients with severe sepsis who are more likely to pass away if otherwise not treated. The debate regarding hemorrhage, a major risk associated with activated protein C, is still ongoing. 3.5% of patients had serious bleeding (intracranial hemorrhage, a life-threatening bleeding episode, or a requirement for 3 or more units of blood), as compared with 2% of patients who received placebo ($P < 0.06$) [29,30].

Therefore, the use of activated protein C is restricted in many hospitals to the more seriously ill patients who meet the criteria for sepsis specified by the Acute Physiology and Chronic Health Evaluation (APACHE II) scoring system.

4. NOVEL THERAPEUTIC STRATEGIES FOR SEPSIS; PIPELINE CANDIDATES

4.1. Immunomodulation

4.1.1. EA-230

EA-230, being developed by Exponential Biotherapies Inc., is a tetrapeptide that has shown renal protective effects in small animal studies [31]. EA-230 acts on the acute kidney injury (AKI) that occurs in almost one-half of patients who develop septic shock [32]. It is being developed for renal protection in septic shock among other conditions, and in experimental studies using the cecal ligation and puncture (CLP) model, EA-230 treatment significantly improved survival in a dose-dependent manner. The best result was obtained with 50 mg/kg EA-230 (43.8% survival after 2 weeks). Serum creatinine and blood urea nitrogen increased markedly 24 h after CLP, and EA-230 significantly attenuated the increases in creatinine and blood urea nitrogen in the 30 to 50 mg/kg treatment groups. Furthermore, the glomerular filtration rate and renal blood flow were significantly higher ($P<0.05$) 36 h post-CLP in EA-230-treated mice versus in those treated with saline [32]. EA-230 is about to enter phase 2 clinical trials following a successful phase 1 study in which the drug was safely tolerated in both single and multiple doses. In this study, EA-230 also attenuated the effects of bacterial lipopolysaccharide administration [33].

4.1.2. TREM-1

TREM (triggering receptor expressed on myeloid cells)-1 is being developed as a decoy receptor by Bioxell SpA and is currently in preclinical trials for the treatment of sepsis. TREM-1 is an activating receptor expressed at high levels on neutrophils and monocytes that infiltrate human tissues infected with bacteria. Furthermore, it is upregulated on peritoneal neutrophils of patients with microbial sepsis and mice with experimental LPS-induced shock [34]. Injection of soluble TREM-1 is able to confer significant protection from mortality in two different preclinical models of sepsis. The survival benefit obtained with the receptor decoy is associated with a significant reduction of the plasma concentrations of inflammatory cytokines. A study on human samples from sepsis patients confirmed the TREM-1 ligand as a diagnostic marker for sepsis. These data indicate that TREM-1 is an important mediator in sepsis and could represent a novel target for therapeutic treatment of the disease [35].

4.2. Coagulation Pathway

4.2.1. LTC-203 (drotrecogin alfa)

Teijin Pharma is conducting phase 1 trials for LTC-203 [drotrecogin alfa activated (DAA) or recombinant human activated protein C], which they have licensed from Eli Lilly. Drotrecogin alfa has many actions including anti-coagulant, anti-inflammatory, and even anti-apoptotic effects [36], and is one of the few interventions that has been shown to improve outcome when administered to patients with severe sepsis [28]. In a previous phase 3 trial, a total of 1690 randomized patients were treated (840 in the placebo group and 850 in the DAA group). The mortality rate was 30.8% in the placebo group and 24.7% in the DAA group. On the basis of the prospectively defined primary analysis, treatment with DAA was associated with a reduction of 19.4% in the relative risk of death (95% confidence interval, 6.6 to 30.5) [28]. Drotrecogin alfa may be targeting the microvascular function by decreasing inflammation and coagulation and increasing fibrinolysis.

In addition to reducing microvascular injury, DAA has been shown to work by improving microcirculatory perfusion [37]. The proportion of perfused capillaries increased in the DAA-treated patients at 4 h (from 64% to 84%, $P<0.01$) but not in the control group (from 67% to 68%, P=not significant) [37]. Microvascular perfusion decreased transiently at the end of drotrecogin alfa infusion. Currently, drotrecogin alfa (Xigris®) is the only FDA-approved therapeutic agent for severe sepsis although the specific mechanisms by which Xigris® exerts its effect on survival in patients with severe sepsis are not completely understood [38].

4.2.2. FX06 / FX107

FX06 is being developed by Fibrex Medical. FX06, a naturally occurring peptide derived from human fibrin, reduces myocardial infarct size in animal models by mitigating reperfusion injury [39]. It binds to vascular endothelial (VE) cadherin, thereby inhibiting tissue inflammation and injury as well as preserving endothelial barrier function.

FX06 reduces infarct size in predictive animal models by a mean of 50%. Preclinical development has been completed. The product is very well tolerated even at very high doses. A proof-of-concept phase 2 trial with Fibrex has recently been completed in patients with acute myocardial infarction undergoing percutaneous coronary intervention (the FIRE study) [40]. In this proof-of-concept trial, FX06 reduced the necrotic core zone as one measure of infarct size on magnetic resonance imaging, while total late enhancement was not significantly different between groups. The drug appears to be safe and well tolerated [39]. FX107, a long-acting derivative for sepsis/septic shock and Dengue shock syndrome, is now in preclinical development.

4.2.3. ATryn®

ATryn® (transgenic antithrombin) is the world's first approved drug that is produced in transgenic goats and is used for the prophylaxis of venous thromboembolism during surgery in patients with congenital antithrombin deficiency. On February 6, 2009, following European Commission approval, the United States Food and Drug Administration announced the approval of ATryn® to treat a rare clotting disorder. ATryn® was first developed by GTC Biotherapeutics, Inc. but LEO pharma A/S has entered into a collaborative agreement to develop and market ATryn® for markets in Europe, the Middle East, and Canada. Estimates from the scientific literature are that there are over 1.5 million cases of severe sepsis in the U.S. and Europe and over 500,000 of these patients develop DIC, with a mortality rate of up to 50% [41-44]. Therefore, from the rationale that explains the relationship between DIC and sepsis, a phase 2 study for severe sepsis is underway. This study, which is currently recruiting participants, will include patients with DIC associated with severe sepsis [45].

4.3. Cell Signaling

4.3.1. E5564

E5564 (Eritoran™), synthesized at Eisai Research Institute of Boston, Inc., is a synthetic analogue of lipid A (toxic component of endotoxin) and is the first TLR4 antagonist to be evaluated in the treatment of severe sepsis. From the IND filing in April 1999, a phase 2 clinical trial for E5564 was completed in April 2005 and a phase 3 trial for sepsis is currently underway [46].

Early preclinical and phase 1 studies have shown that E-5564 administration inhibits LPS-mediated increases in pro-inflammatory cytokine levels and dose-dependently reduces the severity of endotoxin-induced sepsis syndrome in both animal and human models of sepsis [47-49]. In addition, E5564 protected healthy adults from the physiological changes associated with LPS challenge [50]. In agreement with previous studies, the Phase 2 study named "A Safety and Efficacy Study of Intravenous E5564 in Patients with Severe Sepsis" provided optimism for future plans of Eisai. Three hundred patients with early severe sepsis were enrolled in this phase 2 trial, and a double-blind, randomized placebo-controlled staged design study was conducted. E5564 was well-tolerated and transient elevation in the mean value of liver function tests was observed in the high-dose group. In terms of efficacy, high-dose E5564 (105 mg) reduced mortality by 12.2% versus placebo (P=0.09). Moreover, the treatment effect was greater in higher risk patients. The 105-mg group had a 24.8% reduction in mortality versus placebo (P=0.02) [46].

Although efforts to apply E5564 to another disease such as endotoxin-mediated surgical complication were continued, the results were unsuccessful [51]. Recently, Eisai started phase 2 clinical trials for the additional applications for E5564. However, this study was terminated about a month after the start date due to a business decision [52]. The phase 3 clinical trials will determine the effectiveness of TLR4 antagonists in the treatment of patients with severe sepsis.

4.3.2. TAK-242

Since the role of TLR has been unveiled, various approaches are being used to develop TLR agonists and antagonists. TAK-242, one of Takeda's investigational compounds, is a selective antagonist for TLR4, which is known as a representative receptor response to gram-negative infection. Though TAK-242 protected mice against LPS-induced lethality by inhibiting production of multiple cytokines and nitric oxide [53], Takeda discontinued development of this anti-septic agent on February 20, 2009. Reviewing the results from phase 3 clinical trial, TAKEDA concluded that TAK-242's profile did not meet its criteria to support continuation of further development activities.

4.3.3. TBC 1269

TBC 1269 (Bimosiamose) is a pan-selectin antagonist licensed exclusively to Revotar Biopharmaceuticals AG, Henningsdorf, Germany, by Texas Biotechnology Corporation (TBC). TBC's major affiliate Revotar Biopharmaceuticals AG is in phase 2 development of bimosiamose for psoriasis and atopic dermatitis. Sialyl Lewis x glycans [sLe(x)] is a natural ligand for all 3 selectins, which mediate the tethering and rolling of leukocytes on endothelial cells. Several investigations have demonstrated that sLe(x) is a common epitope in many natural selectin ligands, such as P-selectin glycoprotein ligand 1 (PSGL-1), glycosylated cell adhesion molecule 1 (GlyCAM-1), CD34, mucosal addressin cell adhesion molecule 1(MAdCAM-1), and E-selectin ligand 1 (ESL-1) [54]. Due to their low affinity for all three selectins, sLe(x) compounds are potential antagonists for all selectins [55]. Hence, the effort to design the sLe(x)–mimetics has continued. Indeed, one such compound, TBC 1269, was synthesized by Revortar and preclinical studies have demonstrated its anti-inflammatory effects in various species, including rats, sheep, and dogs [56-59]. However, a recent phase 2 clinical trial for asthma failed to show any benefit [60]. Because TBC 1269 has been shown to effectively block selectins in various settings, many researchers have applied this pan-selectin antagonist to other inflammation-related diseases such as endotoxemia. Unfortunately, in 2008, Mayr *et al.* demonstrated that TBC 1269 does not attenuate tissue factor-triggered coagulation or inflammation in human endotoxemia [61].

4.3.4. Anti-HMGB1 mAb

HMGB1 is an abundant protein in nuclei and cytoplasm and is involved in maintaining nucleosome structure and regulating gene transcription [62]. Previous works have demonstrated that HMGB1, a ubiquitous and chromosomal protein, can be actively released from various cells such as RAW 264.7 [63], human primary peripheral blood mononuclear cells [64], and murine erythroleukemia cells [65]. Once released, HMGB1 can bind to cell-surface receptors such as TLR and mediate a variety of cellular responses including chemotactic cell movement and release of pro-inflammatory cytokines [64]. Taken together, these observations characterize HMGB1 as a non-classical, pro-inflammatory cytokine. Moreover, recent evidence suggests that HMGB1 is a late mediator of systemic inflammation [63].

Anti-HMGB1 mAb is a HMGB1-specific neutralizing antibody that is being developed by Critical Therapeutics Inc. Because of its identification as a cytokine, HMGB1 became an attractive candidate mediator for sepsis treatment. In preclinical studies, HMGB1 appears to be a feasible therapeutic target for experimental sepsis [66-68]. However, the clinical application of this mAb is still controversial. In fact, the levels of HMGB1 in unfractionated crude serum of septic patients did not correlate well with disease severity [69,70]. Critical Therapeutics has recently completed preclinical research for this specific amino acid sequence [71].

4.3.5. L-97-1

L-97-1 is a water-soluble small molecule A1 adenosine receptor (A1AR) antagonist with high affinity and high selectivity for the human A1 AR. It is under development in pre-clinical tests as an oral anti-asthma treatment and intravenous sepsis treatment by Endacea, Inc. Previously, in animal model experiments, high-dose L-97-1 (10 mg/kg) blocked early (bronchoconstrictor) and late (inflammatory) allergic responses and bronchial hyper-responsiveness to histamine following house dust mite challenge in an allergic rabbit model of asthma by blocking adenosine A_1 receptors [72]. Endacea is also developing a biomarker for sepsis with POC in humans from a 43-patient pilot clinical trial and optimization studies are in progress [73].

4.3.6. HMGB1 BoxA

Recent structure–function analyses revealed that the DNA-binding domain of HMGB1, the A box, competes with HMGB1 for binding sites on the surface of activated macrophages and attenuates HMGB1-induced release of pro-inflammatory cytokines. Nautilus Biotech and Creabilis Therapeutics entered into collaboration in September 2004 with the aim of developing a usable variant of native HMBG1 Box A with improved pharmacokinetic/ pharmacodynamic characteristics to be used as a direct antagonist of HMGB1 to treat related pathologies including hepatitis B, rheumatoid arthritis, SLE, melanoma, sepsis and MS and/or as an inhibitor of RAGE to treat diabetes complications and inflammatory diseases. Creabilis has completed testing of all the variants, and a limited number of these have increased biological activity *in vitro* and greater resistance to proteolysis. Increased resistance to proteolysis and improved biological activity are important improvements in drug profiles and have the potential to create highly differentiated therapeutic products with better patient compliance.

4.3.7. CT-400

The CT400 program led by Creabilis Therapeutics is aimed at developing inhibitors of HMGB1 to block cell proliferation and migration induced by the protein that is involved in a number of pathologies [74]. CT400, which consists of four DNA strands, is a specific example of the cruciform nucleic acid molecule used to bind the HMGB1 protein [75].

4.4. Endotoxin

4.4.1. IV Alkaline Phosphatase

Hospital-acquired Acute Renal Failure (ARF) occurs in as many as 4% of hospital admissions and 25% of critical care admissions. Mortality from ARF is as high as 50%. ARF can be characterized by elevated serum creatinine levels >150μmol/L (or by rapidly deteriorating serum levels). Alkaline phosphatase (AP) has been shown to reduce serum creatinine levels in ARF patients after AP therapy (24-h infusion). Thus far, AM-Pharma has studied the effects of AP on ARF in sepsis patients [76]. A growing body of evidence suggests that AP plays an important role in host defense in dephosphorylating extracellular ATP [77,78], a known pro-inflammatory molecule, into adenosine, a key molecule in tissue protection mechanisms [79]; extracellular ATP is also involved in the activity of phosphatases and phosphodiesterases [80]. In a phase 2 study with bovine intestinal AP in 36 patients with sepsis and organ failure, the largest organ failure group was "sepsis with acute renal failure (ARF)" (45% of patients). The treatment consisted of a 24-h infusion of AP, which was well tolerated. No drug-related SAEs were reported in the AP group. The all-cause mortality in patients with ARF (controls) was 60% whereas all-cause mortality was 27% in AP-treated patients. However, although all-cause mortality was improved, survival in ARF is dependent on the severity of renal damage for which dialysis (based on creatinine progression, indicator of severity and risk) is the key treatment. Dialysis requirement was reduced from 80% (controls) to 36% (AP-treated patients) in the study.

4.4.2. GR270773

GR270773 is novel phospholipid emulsion derived from a research program by Rogosin and Sepsicure. This compound is designed to bind and remove endotoxin, the most common trigger of the complex series of biochemical and physiologic events that lead to sepsis. The therapeutic rationale for the lipid emulsion developed at Rogosin rests on a natural disease-fighting mechanism. In fact, there are substantial data indicating that serum lipoproteins may neutralize circulating bacterial toxins. High-density lipoprotein (HDL), low-density lipoprotein (LDL), triglyceride-rich lipoproteins, very low density lipoprotein (VLDL), and chylomicron remnants have all been shown to bind and neutralize bacterial endotoxin *in vitro* [81-83]. Previous studies also demonstrated the protective effect of HDL against LPS-induced endotoxemia in both mice and rabbits [84,85]. More recently, infusion of HDL blocked LPS-induced cytokine production in healthy human volunteers and improved cardiopulmonary function and survival in porcine sepsis [86-88].

GlaxoSmithKline completed phase 2 clinical studies in 2006. The phase 2 study was designed as a prospective, randomized, double-blind, placebo-controlled, dose ranging, multi-center study for estimating safety and efficacy of three-day continuous intravenous infusion of GR207003 in suspected or confirmed Gram-negative severe sepsis in adults [89]. According to the announcement from GlaxoSmithKline, neither dose of GR270773 had a beneficial treatment effect on survival or morbidity during the first 28 days of the study. Anemia was the most frequently-reported adverse effect in all groups. Nevertheless, GR270773 is expected to partially improve survival rate in septic patients, and a phase 3 clinical trial is still ongoing.

4.5. Specific Mediators

4.5.1. CytoFab

CytoFab is a polyclonal ovine anti-TNF antigen binding (Fab) fragment that is being developed for the treatment of severe sepsis. CytoFab has been licensed by AstraZeneca, which is responsible for its global development and commercialization in an agreement worth up to 340 million dollars to Protherics in upfront and milestone payments. CytoFab, even smaller anti-TNF-α Fab fragments, effectively reduced serum and BAL TNF-α and serum IL-6 concentrations and increased the number of ventilator-free and ICU-free days at day 28 [90]. At the present time, phase 2 clinical trials are complete for CytoFab, and AstraZeneca's expanded phase 2 program is underway following changes to the manufacturing process, with a 70-patient study due in mid-2009. A second larger study is planned to start shortly thereafter.

4.5.2. NOX-100

NOX-100, also known as Norathiol™, is the first in a series of proprietary small molecule anti-nitric oxide (NO) agents that were created by Medinox. Medinox has finished phase 1/2a clinical trial of NOX-100 in the United States and is planning phase 3 trials.

Medinox announced the clinical results of NOX-100 at the Sixth World Congress on Trauma, Inflammation, Shock and Sepsis in Munich, Germany, on March 3, 2004. The phase 1/2a clinical trial was completed in February, 2004, and fifty-six patients suffering from severe septic shock were enrolled in the double-blind, placebo-controlled multi-center trial. While the 30-day survival rate in patients who received the saline placebo was 42%, the survival rates at 30 days for the NOX-100 groups (by i.v. infusion) were: 1 mg-71%; 3 mg-57%; 6 mg-50%; and 12 mg-63%. All 56 participants who received saline placebo or various NOX-100 doses showed no clinically significant differences in terms of adverse effects [91].

Medinox has agreed to collaborate with Fuso and PUMC Pharmaceutical Co., Ltd., on developing NOX-100. Under the terms of the agreement, Fuso and PUMC are responsible for registration, reimbursement, manufacturing and marketing of NOX-100 in China, South Korea and Japan, respectively [92].

4.5.3. CKD-712

CKD-712, a newly synthesized tetrahydroisoquinoline alkaloid, is being developed by CKD Pharm (Korea) and the phase 1 clinical trial is currently underway in Korea to evaluate its efficacy and safety in sepsis. CKD-712 exerts its pharmacological actions through differential inhibition of iNOS and COX-2 [93]. A previous study reported that YS49, a 1-naphtyl analog of higenamine, has a strong positive inotropic action in isolated rat and rabbit hearts through activation of cardiac β-adrenoceptor [94]. Furthermore, other groups also reported that racemic mixtures of YS49 inhibited iNOS expression and NO production in vascular smooth muscles and RAW 264.7 cells when activated with LPS [95]. CKD712 is an S enantiomer of YS49. Recently, Tsoyi et al. demonstrated differentially regulated LPS-stimulated iNOS and COX-2 production by inhibition of STAT-1 phosphorylation as well as by induction of HO-1 [93].

4.5.4. VX-166

VX-166 is a small molecule caspase inhibitor that was discovered by Vertex. The preclinical study of VX-166 is still ongoing and Vertex Pharmaceuticals holds worldwide rights to VX-166.

Lymphocyte apoptosis contributes to both the onset of sepsis and the progression into septic shock and multiple organ failure [96,97]. When a broad spectrum caspase inhibitor was co-injected with endotoxin, caspase activities and nuclear apoptosis were not only reduced but endotoxin-induced myocardial dysfunction was completely prevented at 4 h and even 14 h after endotoxin challenge [98]. Moreover, using the same caspase inhibitor, Guo et al. demonstrated that caspase inhibition protected against LPS-induced acute renal failure by preventing apoptotic cell death and by inhibiting inflammation [99]. In the preclinical study, VX-166 substantially improved survival in experimental sepsis. In the rat CLP model, 30 mg/kg of VX-166 improved survival from 0% in the vehicle group to 75% in the VX-166 group (P<0.001). At the same time, continuous administration of VX-166 by mini-osmotic pump immediately following CLP improved survival (P<0.01) from 38% in the control group to 88% in the compound-treated group.

Currently, Vertex Pharmaceuticals is considering entering into collaborative arrangements for this drug candidate in order to advance its development [100].

4.5.5. 1-Tetradecanol complex

1-Tetradecanol complex (1-TDC), a novel mono-unsaturated fatty acid mixture, is the first therapeutic drug by Imagenetix (OTCBB:IAGX, San Diego, USA). Initially, application of 1-TDC was mainly focused on the treatment and prevention of periodontal disease. In fact, Imagenetix, Inc., has completed pre-IND assessment by the FDA Dental and Dermatology Division and announced that they received positive comments from the FDA in 2006 [101]. At the present time, Imagenetix is preparing a IND application for 1-TDC, assessing additional studies necessary to meet FDA approval for clinical trials with periodontal diseases and other widespread inflammatory conditions [102].

5. CONCLUSION

The treatment of sepsis is widely regarded as the most challenging problem in intensive care, and presents both clinical and scientific challenges. With only one approved product on the market, Xigris®, sepsis is a renowned graveyard for pipeline candidates. This is partly due to the fact that sepsis is a poorly defined clinical syndrome that encompasses heterogeneous patient populations with potentially diverse disease etiologies. Another substantial issue is that the progression of sepsis is a complex and dynamic pathophysiological process that can lead to either hyperactive or suppressed immune and inflammatory responses, which are still incompletely understood. The majority of the pipeline candidates are currently focused on the systemic response to an infection. While targeting the upstream and the late mediators of sepsis is being emphasized, it is also becoming evident that a more advanced understanding of the precise role of these individual components is essential. Although lowering mortality is the current dominating endpoint, specific strategies that target the pathophysiological disorders in sepsis patients are essential to prevent progression to more severe stages of sepsis and thus further improve clinical outcomes.

REFERENCES

[1]   Marshall, J. C., Deitch, E., Moldawer, L. L., Opal, S., Redl, H., & van der Poll, T. (2005). Preclinical models of shock and sepsis: what can they tell us? Shock, 24 Suppl 1, 1-6.

[2]   Gordon, S. (2002). Pattern recognition receptors: doubling up for the innate immune response. Cell, 111(7), 927-930.

[3]   Armstrong, L., Medford, A. R., Hunter, K. J., Uppington, K. M., & Millar, A. B. (2004). Differential expression of Toll-like receptor (TLR)-2 and TLR-4 on monocytes in human sepsis. Clin Exp Immunol, 136(2), 312-319.

[4]   Tsujimoto, H., Ono, S., Majima, T., Kawarabayashi, N., Takayama, E., Kinoshita, M., Seki, S., Hiraide, H., Moldawer, L. L., & Mochizuki, H. (2005). Neutrophil elastase, MIP-2, and TLR-4 expression during human and experimental sepsis. Shock, 23(1), 39-44.

[5]   Williams, D. L., Ha, T., Li, C., Kalbfleisch, J. H., Schweitzer, J., Vogt, W., & Browder, I. W. (2003). Modulation of tissue Toll-like receptor 2 and 4 during the early phases of polymicrobial sepsis correlates with mortality. Crit Care Med, 31(6), 1808-1818.

[6]   Bouchon, A., Dietrich, J., & Colonna, M. (2000). Cutting edge: inflammatory responses can be triggered by TREM-1, a novel receptor expressed on neutrophils and monocytes. J Immunol, 164(10), 4991-4995.

[7]   Inohara, N., Ogura, Y., & Nunez, G. (2002). Nods: a family of cytosolic proteins that regulate the host response to pathogens. Curr Opin Microbiol, 5(1), 76-80.

[8]   Abbas, A. K., Murphy, K. M., & Sher, A. (1996). Functional diversity of helper T lymphocytes. Nature, 383(6603), 787-793.

[9]   Lolis, E. & Bucala, R. (2003). Therapeutic approaches to innate immunity: severe sepsis and septic shock. Nat Rev Drug Discov, 2(8), 635-645.

[10]   Angstwurm, M., Hoffmann, J., Ostermann, H., Frey, L., & Spannagl, M. (2009). [Severe sepsis and disseminated intravascular coagulation. Supplementation with antithrombin]. Anaesthesist, 58(2), 171-179.

[11]   Michie, H. R., Spriggs, D. R., Manogue, K. R., Sherman, M. L., Revhaug, A., O'Dwyer, S. T., Arthur, K., Dinarello, C. A., Cerami, A., & Wolff, S. M., et al. (1988). Tumor

necrosis factor and endotoxin induce similar metabolic responses in human beings. Surgery, 104(2), 280-286.

[12] Tracey, K. J., Beutler, B., Lowry, S. F., Merryweather, J., Wolpe, S., Milsark, I. W., Hariri, R. J., Fahey, T. J., 3rd, Zentella, A., & Albert, J. D., et al. (1986). Shock and tissue injury induced by recombinant human cachectin. Science, 234(4775), 470-474.

[13] Tracey, K. J., Lowry, S. F., Fahey, T. J., 3rd, Albert, J. D., Fong, Y., Hesse, D., Beutler, B., Manogue, K. R., Calvano, S., & Wei, H., et al. (1987). Cachectin/tumor necrosis factor induces lethal shock and stress hormone responses in the dog. Surg Gynecol Obstet, 164(5), 415-422.

[14] Yang, H., Wang, H., & Tracey, K. J. (2001). HMG-1 rediscovered as a cytokine. Shock, 15(4), 247-253.

[15] Qin, S., Wang, H., Yuan, R., Li, H., Ochani, M., Ochani, K., Rosas-Ballina, M., Czura, C. J., Huston, J. M., Miller, E., Lin, X., Sherry, B., Kumar, A., Larosa, G., Newman, W., Tracey, K. J., & Yang, H. (2006). Role of HMGB1 in apoptosis-mediated sepsis lethality. J Exp Med, 203(7), 1637-1642.

[16] Yu, M., Wang, H., Ding, A., Golenbock, D. T., Latz, E., Czura, C. J., Fenton, M. J., Tracey, K. J., & Yang, H. (2006). HMGB1 signals through toll-like receptor (TLR) 4 and TLR2. Shock, 26(2), 174-179.

[17] Hotchkiss, R. S. & Nicholson, D. W. (2006). Apoptosis and caspases regulate death and inflammation in sepsis. Nat Rev Immunol, 6(11), 813-822.

[18] Cinel, I. & Opal, S. M. (2009). Molecular biology of inflammation and sepsis: a primer. Crit Care Med, 37(1), 291-304.

[19] Deitch, E. A. (1992). Multiple organ failure. Pathophysiology and potential future therapy. Ann Surg, 216(2), 117-134.

[20] Dellinger, R. P., Levy, M. M., Carlet, J. M., Bion, J., Parker, M. M., Jaeschke, R., Reinhart, K., Angus, D. C., Brun-Buisson, C., Beale, R., Calandra, T., Dhainaut, J. F., Gerlach, H., Harvey, M., Marini, J. J., Marshall, J., Ranieri, M., Ramsay, G., Sevransky, J., Thompson, B. T., Townsend, S., Vender, J. S., Zimmerman, J. L., & Vincent, J. L. (2008). Surviving Sepsis Campaign: international guidelines for management of severe sepsis and septic shock: 2008. Crit Care Med, 36(1), 296-327.

[21] Rivers, E., Nguyen, B., Havstad, S., Ressler, J., Muzzin, A., Knoblich, B., Peterson, E., & Tomlanovich, M. (2001). Early goal-directed therapy in the treatment of severe sepsis and septic shock. N Engl J Med, 345(19), 1368-1377.

[22] Rello, J., Ricart, M., Mirelis, B., Quintana, E., Gurgui, M., Net, A., & Prats, G. (1994). Nosocomial bacteremia in a medical-surgical intensive care unit: epidemiologic characteristics and factors influencing mortality in 111 episodes. Intensive Care Med, 20(2), 94-98.

[23] MacArthur, R. D., Miller, M., Albertson, T., Panacek, E., Johnson, D., Teoh, L., & Barchuk, W. (2004). Adequacy of early empiric antibiotic treatment and survival in severe sepsis: experience from the MONARCS trial. Clin Infect Dis, 38(2), 284-288.

[24] Lefering, R. & Neugebauer, E. A. (1995). Steroid controversy in sepsis and septic shock: a meta-analysis. Crit Care Med, 23(7), 1294-1303.

[25] Annane, D., Sebille, V., Charpentier, C., Bollaert, P. E., Francois, B., Korach, J. M., Capellier, G., Cohen, Y., Azoulay, E., Troche, G., Chaumet-Riffaud, P., & Bellissant, E. (2002). Effect of treatment with low doses of hydrocortisone and fludrocortisone on mortality in patients with septic shock. JAMA, 288(7), 862-871.

[26] Abraham, E. & Evans, T. (2002). Corticosteroids and septic shock. JAMA, 288(7), 886-887.

[27] Matthay, M. A. (2001). Severe sepsis--a new treatment with both anticoagulant and antiinflammatory properties. N Engl J Med, 344(10), 759-762.

[28] Bernard, G. R., Vincent, J. L., Laterre, P. F., LaRosa, S. P., Dhainaut, J. F., Lopez-Rodriguez, A., Steingrub, J. S., Garber, G. E., Helterbrand, J. D., Ely, E. W., & Fisher, C. J., Jr. (2001). Efficacy and safety of recombinant human activated protein C for severe sepsis. N Engl J Med, 344(10), 699-709.

[29] Warren, H. S., Suffredini, A. F., Eichacker, P. Q., & Munford, R. S. (2002). Risks and benefits of activated protein C treatment for severe sepsis. N Engl J Med, 347(13), 1027-1030.

[30] Manns, B. J., Lee, H., Doig, C. J., Johnson, D., & Donaldson, C. (2002). An economic evaluation of activated protein C treatment for severe sepsis. N Engl J Med, 347(13), 993-1000.

[31] Goldfarb RD, C. I., Leighton A , Fraimow H, Knob C, Cinel L, Parrillo JE, Dellinger RP. (2008). EA-230 Renal Protection in Porcine Peritonitis. Antimicrobial agents and chemotherapy.

[32] Song Rong, N. S., Jan Menne, Michael Mengel, Paul Leufkens, Michael Brownstein, Hermann Halle, Faikah Gueler. (2008). A novel therapeutic agent to prevent sepsis-induced acute kidney injury and mortality. Critical Care 12(5), 31.

[33] Abraham, E., Anzueto, A., Gutierrez, G., Tessler, S., San Pedro, G., Wunderink, R., Dal Nogare, A., Nasraway, S., Berman, S., Cooney, R., Levy, H., Baughman, R., Rumbak, M., Light, R. B., Poole, L., Allred, R., Constant, J., Pennington, J., & Porter, S. (1998). Double-blind randomised controlled trial of monoclonal antibody to human tumour necrosis factor in treatment of septic shock. NORASEPT II Study Group. Lancet, 351(9107), 929-933.

[34] Bouchon, A., Facchetti, F., Weigand, M. A., & Colonna, M. (2001). TREM-1 amplifies inflammation and is a crucial mediator of septic shock. Nature, 410(6832), 1103-1107.

[35] TREM-1 in Sepsis. (2008). from http://www.bioxell.com/product-pipeline/development-pipeline/inflammatory-diseases/trem-1-in-sepsis/index.lbl

[36] Bernard, G. R. (2003). Drotrecogin alfa (activated) (recombinant human activated protein C) for the treatment of severe sepsis. Crit Care Med, 31(1 Suppl), S85-93.

[37] De Backer, D., Verdant, C., Chierego, M., Koch, M., Gullo, A., & Vincent, J. L. (2006). Effects of drotrecogin alfa activated on microcirculatory alterations in patients with severe sepsis. Crit Care Med, 34(7), 1918-1924.

[38] Mechanism of Action. (2008). from http://www.xigris.com/310-mechanism-of-action.jsp

[39] Atar, D., Petzelbauer, P., Schwitter, J., Huber, K., Rensing, B., Kasprzak, J. D., Butter, C., Grip, L., Hansen, P. R., Suselbeck, T., Clemmensen, P. M., Marin-Galiano, M., Geudelin, B., & Buser, P. T. (2009). Effect of intravenous FX06 as an adjunct to primary percutaneous coronary intervention for acute ST-segment elevation myocardial infarction results of the F.I.R.E. (Efficacy of FX06 in the Prevention of Myocardial Reperfusion Injury) trial. J Am Coll Cardiol, 53(8), 720-729.

[40] Mode of Action_FX06. (2009). from http://www.fibrexmedical.com/technology_2.html

[41] Kohno, S., Inoue, Y., Hayashi, T., Yamaguchi, K., & Hara, K. (1988). Renal insufficiency and DIC in sepsis. Kansenshogaku Zasshi, 62 Suppl, 226-227.

[42] Kambayashi, J., Ogawa, Y., & Kosaki, G. (1983). [Fungal sepsis and DIC in surgical patients]. Nippon Geka Gakkai Zasshi, 84(9), 882-885.

[43] Homola, J. & Prochazka, M. (1980). [Hemolytic anemia and the DIC syndrome in Yersinia sepsis]. Cesk Pediatr, 35(8), 429-431.

[44] Gerjarusak, P., Hinthorn, D. R., & Liu, C. (1977). Hyposplenism and disseminated intravascular coagulation (DIC) in fulminant pneumococcal sepsis. South Med J, 70(8), 995-997.

[45] ATryn. from http://www.clinicaltrials.gov/ct2/show/NCT00506519?term=ATryn% C2%AE &rank=5

[46] News. from http://www.eisai.co.jp/enews/enews200527.html

[47] Czeslick, E., Struppert, A., Simm, A., & Sablotzki, A. (2006). E5564 (Eritoran) inhibits lipopolysaccharide-induced cytokine production in human blood monocytes. Inflamm Res, 55(11), 511-515.

[48] Rossignol, D. P. & Lynn, M. (2002). Antagonism of in vivo and ex vivo response to endotoxin by E5564, a synthetic lipid A analogue. J Endotoxin Res, 8(6), 483-488.

[49] Mullarkey, M., Rose, J. R., Bristol, J., Kawata, T., Kimura, A., Kobayashi, S., Przetak, M., Chow, J., Gusovsky, F., Christ, W. J., & Rossignol, D. P. (2003). Inhibition of endotoxin response by e5564, a novel Toll-like receptor 4-directed endotoxin antagonist. J Pharmacol Exp Ther, 304(3), 1093-1102.

[50] Lynn, M., Wong, Y. N., Wheeler, J. L., Kao, R. J., Perdomo, C. A., Noveck, R., Vargas, R., D'Angelo, T., Gotzkowsky, S., McMahon, F. G., Wasan, K. M., & Rossignol, D. P. (2004). Extended in vivo pharmacodynamic activity of E5564 in normal volunteers with experimental endotoxemia [corrected]. J Pharmacol Exp Ther, 308(1), 175-181.

[51] Bennett-Guerrero, E., Grocott, H. P., Levy, J. H., Stierer, K. A., Hogue, C. W., Cheung, A. T., Newman, M. F., Carter, A. A., Rossignol, D. P., & Collard, C. D. (2007). A phase II, double-blind, placebo-controlled, ascending-dose study of Eritoran (E5564), a lipid A antagonist, in patients undergoing cardiac surgery with cardiopulmonary bypass. Anesth Analg, 104(2), 378-383.

[52] Clinical Trials. from http://clinicaltrials.gov/ct2/show/NCT00756912

[53] Sha, T., Sunamoto, M., Kitazaki, T., Sato, J., Ii, M., & Iizawa, Y. (2007). Therapeutic effects of TAK-242, a novel selective Toll-like receptor 4 signal transduction inhibitor, in mouse endotoxin shock model. Eur J Pharmacol, 571(2-3), 231-239.

[54] Zak, I., Lewandowska, E., & Gnyp, W. (2000). Selectin glycoprotein ligands. Acta Biochim Pol, 47(2), 393-412.

[55] Kogan, T. P., Dupre, B., Keller, K. M., Scott, I. L., Bui, H., Market, R. V., Beck, P. J., Voytus, J. A., Revelle, B. M., & Scott, D. (1995). Rational design and synthesis of small molecule, non-oligosaccharide selectin inhibitors: (alpha-D-mannopyranosyloxy)biphenyl-substituted carboxylic acids. J Med Chem, 38(26), 4976-4984.

[56] Palma-Vargas, J. M., Toledo-Pereyra, L., Dean, R. E., Harkema, J. M., Dixon, R. A., & Kogan, T. P. (1997). Small-molecule selectin inhibitor protects against liver inflammatory response after ischemia and reperfusion. J Am Coll Surg, 185(4), 365-372.

[57] Ramos-Kelly, J. R., Toledo-Pereyra, L. H., Jordan, J., Rivera-Chavez, F., Rohs, T., Holevar, M., Dixon, R. A., Yun, E., & Ward, P. A. (2000). Multiple selectin blockade

with a small molecule inhibitor downregulates liver chemokine expression and neutrophil infiltration after hemorrhagic shock. J Trauma, 49(1), 92-100.

[58] Abraham, W. M., Ahmed, A., Sabater, J. R., Lauredo, I. T., Botvinnikova, Y., Bjercke, R. J., Hu, X., Revelle, B. M., Kogan, T. P., Scott, I. L., Dixon, R. A., Yeh, E. T., & Beck, P. J. (1999). Selectin blockade prevents antigen-induced late bronchial responses and airway hyperresponsiveness in allergic sheep. Am J Respir Crit Care Med, 159(4 Pt 1), 1205-1214.

[59] Cox, C. S., Jr., Allen, S. J., Sauer, H., & Frederick, J. (2000). Effects of selectin-sialyl Lewis blockade on mesenteric microvascular permeability associated with cardiopulmonary bypass. J Thorac Cardiovasc Surg, 119(6), 1255-1261.

[60] Avila, P. C., Boushey, H. A., Wong, H., Grundland, H., Liu, J., & Fahy, J. V. (2004). Effect of a single dose of the selectin inhibitor TBC1269 on early and late asthmatic responses. Clin Exp Allergy, 34(1), 77-84.

[61] Mayr, F. B., Firbas, C., Leitner, J. M., Spiel, A. O., Reiter, R. A., Beyer, D., Meyer, M., Wolff, G., & Jilma, B. (2008). Effects of the pan-selectin antagonist bimosiamose (TBC1269) in experimental human endotoxemia. Shock, 29(4), 475-482.

[62] Goodwin, G. H., Sanders, C., & Johns, E. W. (1973). A new group of chromatin-associated proteins with a high content of acidic and basic amino acids. Eur J Biochem, 38(1), 14-19.

[63] Wang, H., Bloom, O., Zhang, M., Vishnubhakat, J. M., Ombrellino, M., Che, J., Frazier, A., Yang, H., Ivanova, S., Borovikova, L., Manogue, K. R., Faist, E., Abraham, E., Andersson, J., Andersson, U., Molina, P. E., Abumrad, N. N., Sama, A., & Tracey, K. J. (1999). HMG-1 as a late mediator of endotoxin lethality in mice. Science, 285(5425), 248-251.

[64] Andersson, U., Wang, H., Palmblad, K., Aveberger, A. C., Bloom, O., Erlandsson-Harris, H., Janson, A., Kokkola, R., Zhang, M., Yang, H., & Tracey, K. J. (2000). High mobility group 1 protein (HMG-1) stimulates proinflammatory cytokine synthesis in human monocytes. J Exp Med, 192(4), 565-570.

[65] Sparatore, B., Passalacqua, M., Patrone, M., Melloni, E., & Pontremoli, S. (1996). Extracellular high-mobility group 1 protein is essential for murine erythroleukaemia cell differentiation. Biochem J, 320(Pt1), 253-256.

[66] Wang, H., Yang, H., Czura, C. J., Sama, A. E., & Tracey, K. J. (2001). HMGB1 as a late mediator of lethal systemic inflammation. Am J Respir Crit Care Med, 164(10 Pt 1), 1768-1773.

[67] Wang, H., Yang, H., & Tracey, K. J. (2004). Extracellular role of HMGB1 in inflammation and sepsis. J Intern Med, 255(3), 320-331.

[68] Lotze, M. T. & Tracey, K. J. (2005). High-mobility group box 1 protein (HMGB1): nuclear weapon in the immune arsenal. Nat Rev Immunol, 5(4), 331-342.

[69] Sunden-Cullberg, J., Norrby-Teglund, A., Rouhiainen, A., Rauvala, H., Herman, G., Tracey, K. J., Lee, M. L., Andersson, J., Tokics, L., & Treutiger, C. J. (2005). Persistent elevation of high mobility group box-1 protein (HMGB1) in patients with severe sepsis and septic shock. Crit Care Med, 33(3), 564-573.

[70] Angus, D. C., Yang, L., Kong, L., Kellum, J. A., Delude, R. L., Tracey, K. J., & Weissfeld, L. (2007). Circulating high-mobility group box 1 (HMGB1) concentrations are elevated in both uncomplicated pneumonia and pneumonia with severe sepsis. Crit Care Med, 35(4), 1061-1067.

[71] Patent. from http://www.patentstorm.us/patents/7288250.description.html

[72] Obiefuna, P. C., Batra, V. K., Nadeem, A., Borron, P., Wilson, C. N., & Mustafa, S. J. (2005). A novel A1 adenosine receptor antagonist, L-97-1 [3-[2-(4-aminophenyl)-ethyl]-8-benzyl-7-{2-ethyl-(2-hydroxy-ethyl)-amino]-ethyl}-1-propyl-3,7-dihydro-purine-2,6-dione], reduces allergic responses to house dust mite in an allergic rabbit model of asthma. J Pharmacol Exp Ther, 315(1), 329-336.

[73] Endacea, Inc. Product Pipeline. from http://www.endacea.com/pipeline.html

[74] CT 400. (2009). from http://www.creabilistherapeutics.com/projects_8.html

[75] Barone, D. G. (2008). Nucleic Acids For The Treatment Of Hmgb1-Related Pathologies from http://www.freepatentsonline.com/EP1768677.html

[76] Alkaline Phosphatase for treatment of Acute Renal Failure. from http://www.am-pharma.com/download/080730%20rec%20alkaline%20phophatase%20in%20arf%20jul 08.pdf

[77] Ohta, A. & Sitkovsky, M. (2001). Role of G-protein-coupled adenosine receptors in downregulation of inflammation and protection from tissue damage. Nature, 414(6866), 916-920.

[78] Picher, M., Burch, L. H., Hirsh, A. J., Spychala, J., & Boucher, R. C. (2003). Ecto 5'-nucleotidase and nonspecific alkaline phosphatase. Two AMP-hydrolyzing ectoenzymes with distinct roles in human airways. J Biol Chem, 278(15), 13468-13479.

[79] Le Hir, M., Angielski, S., & Dubach, U. C. (1985). Properties of an ecto-5'-nucleotidase of the renal brush border. Ren Physiol, 8(6), 321-327.

[80] Yamane, K. & Maruo, B. (1978). Alkaline phosphatase possessing alkaline phosphodiesterase activity and other phosphodiesterases in Bacillus subtilis. J Bacteriol, 134(1), 108-114.

[81] Freudenberg, M. A., Bog-Hansen, T. C., Back, U., & Galanos, C. (1980). Interaction of lipopolysaccharides with plasma high-density lipoprotein in rats. Infect Immun, 28(2), 373-380.

[82] Harris, H. W., Grunfeld, C., Feingold, K. R., Read, T. E., Kane, J. P., Jones, A. L., Eichbaum, E. B., Bland, G. F., & Rapp, J. H. (1993). Chylomicrons alter the fate of endotoxin, decreasing tumor necrosis factor release and preventing death. J Clin Invest, 91(3), 1028-1034.

[83] Ulevitch, R. J., Johnston, A. R., & Weinstein, D. B. (1981). New function for high density lipoproteins. Isolation and characterization of a bacterial lipopolysaccharide-high density lipoprotein complex formed in rabbit plasma. J Clin Invest, 67(3), 827-837.

[84] Levine, D. M., Parker, T. S., Donnelly, T. M., Walsh, A., & Rubin, A. L. (1993). In vivo protection against endotoxin by plasma high density lipoprotein. Proc Natl Acad Sci U S A, 90(24), 12040-12044.

[85] Hubsch, A. P., Powell, F. S., Lerch, P. G., & Doran, J. E. (1993). A reconstituted, apolipoprotein A-I containing lipoprotein reduces tumor necrosis factor release and attenuates shock in endotoxemic rabbits. Circ Shock, 40(1), 14-23.

[86] Pajkrt, D., Lerch, P. G., van der Poll, T., Levi, M., Illi, M., Doran, J. E., Arnet, B., van den Ende, A., ten Cate, J. W., & van Deventer, S. J. (1997). Differential effects of reconstituted high-density lipoprotein on coagulation, fibrinolysis and platelet activation during human endotoxemia. Thromb Haemost, 77(2), 303-307.

[87] Pajkrt, D., Doran, J. E., Koster, F., Lerch, P. G., Arnet, B., van der Poll, T., ten Cate, J. W., & van Deventer, S. J. (1996). Antiinflammatory effects of reconstituted high-density lipoprotein during human endotoxemia. J Exp Med, 184(5), 1601-1608.

[88] Goldfarb, R. D., Parker, T. S., Levine, D. M., Glock, D., Akhter, I., Alkhudari, A., McCarthy, R. J., David, E. M., Gordon, B. R., Saal, S. D., Rubin, A. L., Trenholme, G. M., & Parrillo, J. E. (2003). Protein-free phospholipid emulsion treatment improved cardiopulmonary function and survival in porcine sepsis. Am J Physiol Regul Integr Comp Physiol, 284(2), R550-557.

[89] GR270773. from http://www.gsk-clinicalstudyregister.com/protocol_comp_list.jsp?compound=Gr270773

[90] Rice, T. W., Wheeler, A. P., Morris, P. E., Paz, H. L., Russell, J. A., Edens, T. R., & Bernard, G. R. (2006). Safety and efficacy of affinity-purified, anti-tumor necrosis factor-alpha, ovine fab for injection (CytoFab) in severe sepsis. Crit Care Med, 34(9), 2271-2281.

[91] NOX-100. from http://www.medinox.com/home/articles/7/index.html

[92] NOX-100 News. from http://www.biospace.com/news_story.aspx?NewsEntityId=17104020

[93] Tsoyi, K., Kim, H. J., Shin, J. S., Kim, D. H., Cho, H. J., Lee, S. S., Ahn, S. K., Yun-Choi, H. S., Lee, J. H., Seo, H. G., & Chang, K. C. (2008). HO-1 and JAK-2/STAT-1 signals are involved in preferential inhibition of iNOS over COX-2 gene expression by newly synthesized tetrahydroisoquinoline alkaloid, CKD712, in cells activated with lipopolysacchride. Cell Signal, 20(10), 1839-1847.

[94] Lee, Y. S., Kim, C. H., Yun-Choi, H. S., & Chang, K. C. (1994). Cardiovascular effect of a naphthylmethyl substituted tetrahydroisoquinoline, YS 49, in rat and rabbit. Life Sci, 55(21), PL415-420.

[95] Kang, Y. J., Koo, E. B., Lee, Y. S., Yun-Choi, H. S., & Chang, K. C. (1999). Prevention of the expression of inducible nitric oxide synthase by a novel positive inotropic agent, YS 49, in rat vascular smooth muscle and RAW 264.7 macrophages. Br J Pharmacol, 128(2), 357-364.

[96] Hotchkiss, R. S., Coopersmith, C. M., & Karl, I. E. (2005). Prevention of lymphocyte apoptosis--a potential treatment of sepsis? Clin Infect Dis, 41 Suppl 7, S465-469.

[97] Hotchkiss, R. S., Osmon, S. B., Chang, K. C., Wagner, T. H., Coopersmith, C. M., & Karl, I. E. (2005). Accelerated lymphocyte death in sepsis occurs by both the death receptor and mitochondrial pathways. J Immunol, 174(8), 5110-5118.

[98] Neviere, R., Fauvel, H., Chopin, C., Formstecher, P., & Marchetti, P. (2001). Caspase inhibition prevents cardiac dysfunction and heart apoptosis in a rat model of sepsis. Am J Respir Crit Care Med, 163(1), 218-225.

[99] Guo, R., Wang, Y., Minto, A. W., Quigg, R. J., & Cunningham, P. N. (2004). Acute renal failure in endotoxemia is dependent on caspase activation. J Am Soc Nephrol, 15(12), 3093-3102.

[100] Vertex Pharmaceuticals. from http://apps.shareholder.com/sec/viewerContent.aspx?companyid=VRTX&docid=5003347

[101] Imagenetix. from http://www.imagenetix.net/articles/206/007_06.php

[102] 1-TDC. from http://www.imagenetix.net/articles/2006/05_06.php

In: Sepsis: Symptoms, Diagnosis and Treatment
Editor: Joseph R. Brown, pp. 75-92

ISBN: 978-1-60876-609-3
© 2010 Nova Science Publishers, Inc.

Chapter 4

THE LIPEMIA OF SEPSIS: TRIGLYCERIDE-RICH LIPOPROTEINS AS AGENTS OF INNATE IMMUNITY

Kelley I. Chuang and Hobart W. Harris
University of California San Francisco, California, USA

ABSTRACT

Bacterial endotoxin (i.e., lipopolysaccharide [LPS]) elicits dramatic responses in the host, including elevated plasma lipid levels due to increased synthesis and secretion of triglyceride-rich lipoproteins by the liver and inhibition of lipoprotein lipase. This cytokine-induced hyperlipoproteinemia, clinically termed the "lipemia of sepsis," was customarily thought to involve the mobilization of lipid stores to fuel the host response to infection. However, because lipoproteins can also bind and neutralize LPS, we have long postulated that triglyceride-rich lipoproteins (very-low-density lipoproteins and chylomicrons) are also components of an innate, nonadaptive host immune response to infection. Once the lipid A portion of LPS inserts into the accepting lipoprotein, its ability to stimulate LPS-responsive cells is diminished whereas its catabolism is increased. Furthermore, hepatic metabolism of lipoprotein-bound LPS results in an attenuated response of hepatocytes to proinflammatory cytokines, a process termed "cytokine tolerance." Several studies have shown that elevated plasma lipoprotein levels are protective against LPS-mediated toxicity in vertebrates. Recent studies have shown that apolipoprotein E, a component of plasma lipoproteins, is a key mediator of immunoregulation. Exogenous administration of apolipoprotein E increases mortality in a murine model of sepsis. Apolipoprotein E acts as a molecular chaperone for bacterial antigens, resulting in downstream Natural Killer T cell activation and cytokine secretion. Insight into the mechanism of lipoprotein-mediated immunomodulation has opened the door to potential novel treatment strategies of sepsis.

INTRODUCTION

Among the various changes that occur when animals or humans are challenged with infectious agents or endotoxin (i.e., lipopolysaccharide [LPS]) is a significant alteration in the distribution of their circulating lipoproteins. This clinical condition, termed the "lipemia of sepsis," was initially described in 1959, when patients with cholera were noted to have grossly lipemic blood and high serum levels of triglyceride[1]. The same observations were noted in patients experiencing polymicrobial infection [2], and the phenomenon has since been sporadically described in the literature. Experimental studies have shown that the lipemia of sepsis is primarily due to the accumulation of very-low-density lipoproteins, although levels of other lipid moieties, including glycerol, triglycerides, and fatty acids, are also elevated (Table 1)[3].

Our understanding of the mechanism underlying the lipemia of sepsis is evolving. Studies suggest that, after an infectious challenge, catabolism of circulating lipoproteins decreases, and lipoprotein production increases [4, 5]. While specific effector molecules that trigger these alterations have not yet been completely elucidated, several theories have been proposed. In the mid-1980s, the lipemia induced by LPS was suggested to be secondary to the release of cachectin, or tumor necrosis factor (TNF) [6-8]. Administration of TNF, already known to mimic the physiological effects of LPS, increased the mobilization of stored body fat and increased turnover of free fatty acids [9]. But this theory was questioned when, in the early 1990s, anti-TNF antibodies did not prevent lipemia in LPS-treated rats. A second theory suggested that the LPS-induced lipemia was an effect of adrenergic stimulation [10]. Nongaki et al. found that α–adrenergic blockade, but not β- adrenergic blockade, resulted in the absence of LPS-induced lipemia, suggesting a non-TNF-mediated process. Currently, the lipemia of sepsis is thought to be a complex integrated response regulated by both the cytokines and the sympathetic nervous system, befitting a system integral to host survival.

Both cytokine and α–adrenergic stimulation appear to alter the activity of several lipolytic enzymes. For example, gram-negative infection has been shown in rodents to attenuate the activity of lipoprotein lipase in adipose tissue. Lipoprotein lipase is critical to hepatic lipid metabolism because once fatty acids reach the liver, they can either be oxidized as an immediate energy source or re-esterified to very-low-density lipoprotein (VLDL) trigylcerides and redistributed throughout the body. Since lipoprotein lipase cleaves fatty acids from the triacylglycerols its inhibition results in a decreased ability to catabolize and thus clear circulating triglycerides [11, 12]. Interestingly, the effect of LPS on lipid metabolism is dose-dependent. Low dose LPS (100 ng/100g body weight) produces hyperlipidemia through stimulation of de novo hepatic fatty acid synthesis and lipolysis. The hyperlipidemia following high dose LPS (50 µg/100g body weight) is due to decreased lipoprotein lipase activity and triglyceride (TG)-rich lipoprotein clearance by the liver [13].

Hormone-sensitive lipase is another important lipolytic enzyme stimulated by systemic signals. The enzyme is activated in adipose tissue following LPS challenge and, like lipoprotein lipase, liberates fatty acids from circulating lipoproteins for uptake by the liver and skeletal muscle. A variety of hormones and growth factors regulate hormone-sensitive lipase. In adipose tissue, the enzyme is inhibited by insulin and stimulated by catecholamines, cortisol and growth hormone. In addition to these lipolytic enzymes, cytokines and LPS also affect the activity of fatty acyl CoA synthetase, which catalyzes the conversion of long-chain fatty acids to esters. LPS and cytokines have been shown to increase fatty acyl CoA synthetase activity in mitochondria, resulting in re-esterification of free fatty acids for trigylceride production [10]. While our understanding of the inter-related effects of cytokines and the adrenergic nervous system on lipid metabolism is incomplete, the neuroendocrine response to infection clearly includes the elevation of plasma lipid levels. As noted above, this hyperlipidemia may simply represent the mobilization of energy stores to fuel the increased metabolic demands of the host. However, the capacity of lipoproteins to directly interact with bacterial, viral and fungal toxins certainly raises the possibility that these particles may function as more than lipid transporters.

In the past decade, considerable interest has focused on the innate immune response and the various components of this more primitive arm of the immune system. Here we review findings emerging from current research and highlight an underappreciated link between innate immune defense mechanisms and lipid metabolism. The cytokine-mediated production of triglyceride-rich lipoproteins observed during states of acute stress and injury has prompted the hypothesis that lipoproteins are components of the host response to infection. Substantial evidence now indicates that not only do triglyceride-rich lipoproteins bind and neutralize LPS, but that lipoprotein-LPS complexes can exert an immunomodulatory effect on cells critical to host immune defenses.

LIPOPROTEINS BIND ENDOTOXIN

The hypothesis that triglyceride-rich lipoproteins are components of an innate host immune response to infection results largely from observations made while studying chylomicron metabolism in humans in 1988. At that time, chylomicron-enriched plasma samples were noted to contain large quantities of LPS (>10 pg of LPS/mg of lipoprotein triglyceride), which was undetected by the standard Limulus assay [14, 15]. Numerous plasma proteins can inhibit the Limulus assay, but, because LPS also increases the production of triglyceride-rich lipoproteins by the liver, it was only natural to question whether these two observations might not be indicative of coordinated facets of a physiological defense mechanism.

Table 1. Effect of Gram-negative sepsis on lipid metabolism as shown by concentrations of glycerol, triglycerides and non-esterified fatty acids

	Glycerol (μM)	Triglycerides (μM)	Fatty acids (μM)
Control	70	1250	970
Septic	130	5020	6450

The data in this table were derived from Samra et al. [3]

Until the late 1980s, most of the work examining the interaction between lipoproteins and LPS focused on the cholesterol ester–rich high-density and low-density lipoproteins. Ulevitch et al. demonstrated the ability of high density lipoprotein (HDL) to bind LPS as part of a two-step process requiring serum [16-18]. This work showed that initially, serum appeared to disaggregate macromolecules of LPS, and that subsequently, the disaggregated LPS binds to HDL, as evidenced by a decrease in the buoyant density of LPS when ultracentrifuged in a CsCl gradient. Ulevitch et al. further demonstrated that once LPS was bound to high-density lipoproteins, its ability to induce fever, leukocytosis, and hypotension was dramatically reduced [16, 17]. The binding of LPS to high-density lipoproteins also prevented endotoxin-induced death in mice that had undergone an adrenalectomy [16]. Van Lenten et al. demonstrated that low-density lipoprotein (LDL) could also bind LPS in much the same way [19]. LPS bound to LDL showed less toxicity to endothelial cells, although it could initiate some components of the inflammatory response [20]. Importantly, previous studies that examined a potential interaction between triglyceride-rich lipoproteins and LPS had shown that VLDL had much less ability to interact and form complexes with LPS than did the cholesterol-rich low- and high-density lipoproteins [17, 19]. In fact, one study suggested that the reason for this difference might be that a lipoprotein's ability to interact with LPS is directly proportional to its cholesterol content [19]. In support of this conclusion, the investigators demonstrated that LPS binding was substantially increased in the triglyceride-rich lipoprotein fraction from Watanabe heritable hyperlipidemic and cholesterol-fed rabbits as compared to controls. In these hyperlipidemic animals, the triglyceride-rich lipoprotein fraction contained the cholesterol-enriched β–VLDL rather than the relatively cholesterol-poor VLDL present in the normolipidemic animals. The interaction of chylomicron with LPS had not yet been examined.

Subsequently, it has been conclusively demonstrated that all lipoproteins can bind and neutralize the toxic effects of LPS, both in vitro [14] and in vivo [21]. Very-low-density lipoproteins and chylomicron have been shown to effectively protect mice against LPS-induced death. In addition, a commercially available triglyceride-rich lipid emulsion used for parenteral nutrition in humans (Soyacal) also protected mice from LPS-induced toxicity [21]. Because all of these lipid particles are large and rich in triglyceride, and contain little, or, in the case of the lipid emulsion, no cholesterol, these results demonstrated that cholesterol was not essential or necessary for the interaction between lipoproteins and LPS to take place. Furthermore, the protective ability of all lipoproteins tested, including low-density lipoproteins and high-density lipoproteins, was directly dependent on the concentration of lipoprotein phospholipid present in the endotoxin-lipoprotein mixtures [22, 23].

The principles of classic receptor-ligand binding do not govern the interaction between lipoproteins and LPS, because there is no LPS receptor on the surface of lipoproteins. Rather, LPS is thought to simply dissolve into the phospholipid coat of the lipid particle. The nature of the lipoprotein-LPS binding process thus predicts that the lipid A moiety is the region of the LPS macromolecule that inserts into the phospholipid monolayer of the lipoprotein. The lipid A–phospholipid interaction effectively reduces the bioavailability of LPS and thus neutralizes its toxic effects. The observation that all classes of lipoproteins and a synthetic lipid emulsion could protect against endotoxicity led us to presume that a lipid-glycolipid interaction must be at least partially responsible for this phenomenon [21]. Subsequent to our initial observations, Parker et al. [23] examined the capacity of various lipoproteins and lipid particles to bind LPS from both smooth- and rough-type gram-negative bacteria and, through a stepwise linear regression analysis of particle composition, found that only phospholipid content was correlated with effectiveness. The concept that the phospholipid content of a lipid particle determines its capacity to bind and neutralize LPS is also supported by findings that reconstituted high-density lipoprotein preparations with the highest phospholipid content yielded the greatest degree of protection in an in vivo model of sepsis [22].

SERUM PROTEINS REGULATE LIPOPROTEIN-LPS INTERACTIONS

It has been recognized for more than 20 years that the interaction between LPS and lipoproteins is dependent on plasma factors [24, 25]. Although several plasma proteins can interact with LPS, none have been more extensively studied than CD14 [26] and the acute-phase reactant LPS-binding protein (LBP) [27, 28]. Together, these two proteins dramatically affect both the sensitivity and overall magnitude of the host response to LPS.

CD14, a 55 kDa glycoprotein originally described in 1982 [29], has been idenitified as an important LPS effector molecule. Expressed on the surface of monocytes and macrophages at up to 50,000 molecules/cell [29], the first indication that CD14 functions as an LPS receptor came from studies in which anti-CD14 antibodies selectively prevented macrophage binding to LPS-coated erythrocytes [25]. It now appears that CD14 acts in combination with LBP as part of a high-affinity LPS recognition mechanism, facilitating macrophage activation by picogram quantities of LPS [21]. LPS and LBP appear to form a complex in serum in which LPS is subsequently transferred to CD14 before the toxic macromolecule ultimately triggers an intracellular signal. Exactly how LPS binding to CD14 initiates an intracellular signal cascade is not clear, especially because the protein lacks a transmembrane domain [30]. Binding studies showed that monoclonal antibodies that block CD14 can only partially inhibit LPS-binding, which suggests that additional transmembrane receptors work in conjunction with LPS-CD14 to initiate the signaling process [31-33]. CD14 exists in two forms: one form is expressed by macrophages and by other myeloid lineage cells and is anchored to the cell membrane through a glycosylphosphatidylinositol (GPI) linkage (mCD14);,the other form is soluble (sCD14). The soluble form of CD14 was originally described in 1985 due to its ability to block the staining of monocytes with anti-CD14 monoclonal antibody [34]. Present in the serum of normal individuals at a concentration of 4-6 µg/ml [35], this 50-53 kDa glycoprotein enables various cells which do not express mCD14 to respond to low doses of LPS, including endothelial and epithelial cells [36, 37]. Apparently, these nonmyeloid cells have a protein on their surface that recognizes CD14-LPS complexes, as evidenced by non-denaturing polyacrylamide gel electrophoresis analysis and the ability to inhibit the serum-dependent, LPS-mediated activation of endothelial cells via immunodepletion of CD14 [38-40]. Although important aspects of LPS-induced cellular activation are currently unknown, CD14 undoubtedly plays a central role in the pathogenesis of gram-negative sepsis.

Despite the initial prominence assigned to CD14, considerable evidence indicates that LBP also plays a significant role in the host response to LPS. In fact, LBP likely assumes an equally important function in the recognition and catabolism of circulating LPS. Endotoxins are amphipathic molecules that readily form micellar aggregates within aqueous environments. These aggregates react very poorly with leukocytes and thus provoke very little in the way of a cellular response. LBP and soluble CD14 are two plasma proteins that dramatically enhance the host response to LPS [41]. LBP is a 60-kDa class 1 acute-phase protein secreted by the liver in response to injury, trauma, or infection. In addition, LBP shares structural and functional homology with a family of lipid transfer proteins (i.e., cholesterol ester transfer protein and phospholipid transfer protein), and a bactericidal leukocyte granule protein termed bactericidal/permeability-increasing protein [42-44]. Like CD14, LBP participates in the binding and transfer of LPS from micellar aggregates [45, 46], bacterial membranes [47], and mononuclear cells [48] to lipoproteins and other phospholipids or cell membranes (Figure 1). Specifically, LBP is thought to facilitate the binding of monomeric LPS by CD14 (membrane-bound and soluble forms) and thus promote LPS-induced cellular activation. Thus, circulating LPS may first react with LBP and in so doing define a core role for this acute-phase reactant in the host response to gram-negative sepsis. The relative contribution of LBP versus CD14 to the catabolism of LPS remains the subject of intense research, but clearly both proteins are essential to the binding of LPS by plasma lipoproteins [38, 48, 49] and thus integral components of the innate immune response to infection.

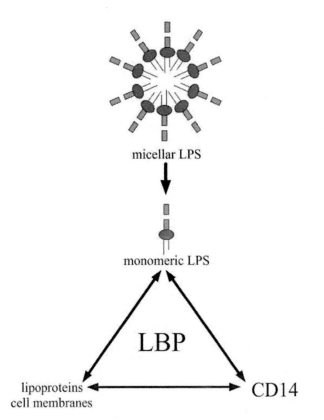

Figure 1. Transfer reactions promoted by lipopolysaccharide (LPS)-binding protein (LBP). LBP facilitates the transfer of monomeric LPS from micellar aggregates to both membrane-bound and soluble CD14. In addition, LBP can directly transfer LPS to lipoproteins

LIPOPROTEINS PROTECT AGAINST ENDOTOXIN

Central to the hypothesis that triglyceride-rich lipoproteins are components of an innate, non-adaptive host immune response to infection is their increased synthesis and secretion during sepsis and their capacity to protect against LPS-induced toxicity and death. Early evidence of the protective effect of lipoprotein binding on LPS toxicity came from the work of Ulevitch *et al.* [16, 17], who showed that in mice, the capacity of high-density lipoprotein–bound LPS to induce fever, leukocytosis, hypotension, and death was dramatically reduced, compared with that of LPS alone. Our laboratory also used a murine model of sepsis to show that all lipoproteins, along with a synthetic triglyceride-rich lipid emulsion, could protect against LPS-induced lethality [21]. Furthermore, we presented data supporting a role for endogenous triglyceride-rich lipoproteins in the sequestration and neutralization of LPS *in vivo* in humans [50].

Additional evidence supporting a protective role for lipoproteins against endotoxicity has emerged over the past several years. Different experimental models have been used, but each study shared the underlying hypothesis that elevated plasma lipoprotein levels are protective against LPS-mediated toxicity in vertebrates. In all of these studies, hyperlipoproteinemia was induced by one of the following: the infusion of exogenous lipoproteins [51, 52], synthetic emulsions [21, 52], or recombinant lipoproteins [22-24, 53-56]; genetic manipulation of the catabolic machinery for lipoproteins [38, 57]; or diet [58]. Regardless of the method for inducing hyperlipoproteinemia, elevations in the circulating level of any class of lipoprotein afforded protection against LPS, compared with effects in normolipidemic controls. Furthermore, hypolipidemic animals have an increased susceptibility to the toxicity of LPS that is reversed when plasma lipid levels return to the normal range [51].

Most of the evidence supporting a protective role for lipoproteins against LPS has understandably been generated with animal models of infection. Few studies have examined this question in humans, and the existing data are contradictory and thus inconclusive. van der Poll *et al.* [59] examined the effect of hypertriglyceridemia on the response to LPS in humans. Although a triglyceride-rich fat emulsion inhibited LPS-induced cytokine production in human whole blood in vitro, concurrent in vivo studies yielded the opposite conclusion. To examine the in vivo effects, volunteers were given a bolus injection of purified LPS (4 ng/kg; lot EC-5) halfway through an infusion of either a triglyceride-rich emulsion or dextrose 5% (controls). The lipid infusion produced significant hypertriglyceridemia, yet the elevated lipid levels did not reduce the LPS-induced fever, leukocytosis, or TNF-α release compared with that measured in the control group. In addition, the lipid infusion apparently potentiated specific LPS responses, including the production of IL-6 and IL-8, neutrophil degranulation, and activation of the coagulation system [56]. Precisely what accounts for these discrepant results is not known. However, differences between the metabolism of lipoproteins versus lipid emulsions [60-63] and the kinetics of LPS binding by triglyceride-rich lipoproteins may, in part, be responsible [21, 49]. The catabolism of triglyceride-rich fat emulsions is complex and includes the generation of phospholipid-rich discoid particles termed lipoprotein-X. These abnormal lipid particles not only interfere with the clearance of endogenous triglyceride-rich lipoproteins [64], they also have a prolonged circulating half-life measured in days (24-60 hr) [65], rather than the minutes required for the clearance of chylomicron or VLDL. Accordingly, LPS bound to lipoprotein-X would be expected to remain in the circulation for days where it would be potentially available to activate cellular and non-cellular components of the immune system for an extended period. In addition, clinically relevant exposures to LPS in humans are likely to be more gradual than the abrupt bolus exposures examined in the van der Poll study.

Another important variable to consider regarding the protective capacity of lipoproteins is the kinetics of lipoprotein-LPS binding. This process is relatively slow, compared with the binding of LPS by leukocytes [23, 49]. Consequently, we have customarily preincubated the lipoproteins and LPS together before administration to specifically facilitate their interaction [21, 66, 67]. In so doing, we selectively study the cellular or host response to lipoprotein-LPS complexes and not the kinetics of binding. The study design used by van der Poll et al. [59] to study the effect of hypertriglyceridemia on the response to LPS necessarily examined both the kinetics of binding and the host response to LPS simultaneously. In contrast, our laboratory has examined the effect of triglyceride-rich lipoproteins on the response to LPS in humans by following an experimental protocol modeled after our rodent studies. In these studies, we have shown that both fasting and postprandial lipoproteins can inhibit the effects of LPS in humans [50]. Volunteers infused with LPS (4 ng/kg) that had been preincubated with either fasting or postprandial whole human blood had lower maximal temperatures, leukocyte counts, and plasma adrenocorticotropic hormone and TNF-α levels than did controls injected with LPS in saline. Although the overall clinical utility of lipids to combat gram-negative infections remains an open question, these findings in humans clearly parallel the results from numerous animal studies.

Therefore, on the basis of current information, lipoproteins modulate the host response to endotoxin by inhibiting the activation of macrophages, monocytes, and other LPS-responsive cells, promoting the catabolism of LPS by the hepatic parenchymal cells, and inhibiting the response of hepatocytes to proinflammatory stimuli. Once introduced into the circulation, monomeric LPS is transferred to phospholipid-rich membranes through the action of LBP and CD14. The transfer or "binding" process appears to involve the actual insertion of the lipid A domain of LPS into the phospholipid leaflet of the accepting cellular membrane or lipoprotein's surface coat. Because the lipophilic lipid A domain of the macromolecule is almost exclusively responsible for the toxic effects of LPS, the transfer process effectively masks this region, thereby reducing its bioavailability. As has been predicted, lipoprotein-bound LPS, with its lipid A domain rendered biologically invisible, is significantly less stimulatory to macrophages [67], monocytes [68-70] and other LPS-sensitive tissues.

Lipemia of Sepsis

The molecular basis for the lipemia of sepsis is only beginning to be understood. In our effort to tease apart this complex integration between the host immune system and lipid metabolism, we have focused on the capacity of chylomicron and VLDL to neutralize LPS and thus protect against endotoxic shock and death in rodent models of sepsis [21, 66]. Early in the course of this work, we found that chylomicron increases the clearance of LPS by the liver while decreasing overall TNF-α production. The binding of LPS to chylomicron more than doubled the amount of endotoxin taken up by the liver, with most of the increased clearance observed due to uptake of the microbial toxin by hepatocytes rather than by Kupffer cells [67]. The internalized LPS significantly attenuated the response of hepatocytes to proinflammatory cytokines. On the basis of these findings, we hypothesized that triglyceride-rich lipoproteins are components of an innate host immune response to infection and that the hepatic metabolism of triglyceride-rich lipoproteins is part of a cytokine-mediated host homeostatic mechanism (Figure 2). Specifically, when animals are exposed to LPS, there is a cytokine-mediated increase in the hepatic synthesis and secretion of triglyceride-rich lipoproteins that, when released, act to "scavenge" for circulating LPS. The resultant lipoprotein-bound LPS is then taken up by hepatocytes. Once internalized, the lipoprotein-bound LPS transiently attenuates the response of hepatocytes to circulating proinflammatory cytokines (a process termed "cytokine tolerance"), thereby down-regulating the overall acute phase response. Currently, we are studying the molecular mechanism behind this potentially novel biological observation, including how chylomicron-LPS complexes interact with hepatocytes to subsequently attenuate their response to cytokines. We are also exploring the possibility that any cell capable of the receptor-mediated internalization of lipoprotein-bound LPS will also assume a cytokine-tolerant phenotype. These most recent studies are focused on cells that express the low-density lipoprotein receptor and are critical to the innate immune response to infection, including adrenocortical cells and vascular endothelial cells. Knowledge of how lipoprotein-bound LPS influences the activation of cytoplasmic signaling molecules within various epithelial cells is crucial to our understanding of the host response to infection.

Utilizing an in vitro system, we have confirmed and extended the in vivo observations showing that chylomicron-LPS complexes can exert an anti-inflammatory effect on hepatocytes [67]. Recent data demonstrate that the pretreatment of hepatocytes with chylomicron-bound LPS attenuates nitric oxide (NO) production by dampening cytokine-induced NF-κB activation. Hepatocytes pretreated with chylomicron-LPS complexes exhibit a significant reduction in cytokine-induced NO production [71]. Neither LPS nor chylomicron alone have any significant effect on NO production, yet the combination reduces the detectable nitrite yield by approximately 60%. Since chylomicron-bound LPS pretreatment attenuates the response of hepatocytes to a combination of different cytokines, we postulated that NF-κB, a transcription factor known to be activated by pro-inflammatory cytokines, might represent the potential site of inhibition. We then demonstrated that chylomicron-LPS complexes can inhibit the cytokine-induced activation of NF-κB in rat hepatocytes. Specifically, cells pretreated with chylomicron-LPS contained significantly less activated NF-KB than did cells pretreated with either LPS or chylomicron alone.

Since endothelial cells are integral to the immune response and similarly express LDLRs, we repeated a similar set of experiments looking at cytokine tolerance in vascular endothelial cells [unpublished data]. Rat postcapillary mesenteric venules were treated with TNF-α and PAF and capillary leak was measured using the Landis microcannulation technique. We found that chylomicron-LPS complexes attenuated cytokine-induced hydraulic conductivity. In addition, nuclear and cytoplasmic levels of p65 were reduced after TNF-α stimulation in endothelial cell monolayers pretreated with chylomicron-LPS, a finding consistent with inhibition of NF-κB translocation.

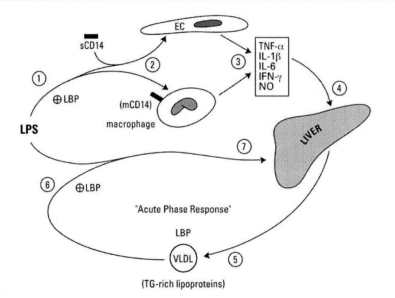

Figure 2. Proposed modulation of the host inflammatory response by triglyceride (TG)-rich lipoproteins. Once endotoxin (LPS) enters the circulation *(1)*, it rapidly stimulates macrophages (myeloid) and endothelial (nonmyeloid) cells (EC) *(2)* to produce numerous soluble mediators of inflammation *(3)*, including TNF-α, IL-1β, and nitric oxide (NO). LPS triggers cell activation through a variety of proteins, including LPS-binding protein (LBP) and membrane-bound CD14 (mCD14) and soluble CD14 (sCD14). Interestingly, the liver is not directly stimulated by circulating LPS, but is instead activated by the cytokine products of LPS-responsive cells *(4)*. Consequently, the liver responds to the endotoxic challenge with a dramatic alteration in hepatic protein synthesis termed "the acute-phase response." This cytokine-mediated change in gene expression includes the increased production and release of TG-rich lipoproteins (VLDL) and LBP *(5)*, a 60-kDa protein with lipid transfer activity capable of "binding" LPS to lipoproteins *(6)*. We postulate that TG-rich lipoproteins modulate the host response to LPS, first by the formation of lipoprotein-LPS complexes that "scavenge" the LPS still remaining in the circulation, thus neutralizing its toxicity, and second, by the complexes being cleared by the liver *(7)* in a manner that dampens the hepatic response to further cytokine stimulation, thereby modulating the acute-phase response.

Collectively, these findings show that chylomicron-bound LPS exerts an inhibitory effect on the cytokine-induced activation of NF-κB in rat hepatocytes and vascular endothelial cells. The anti-inflammatory effect of chylomicron-LPS complexes likely represents an endogenous mechanism by which the host regulates the hepatic acute phase response and the endothelial response to cytokines. These findings also indicate that LPS may both initiate and regulate the host inflammatory response to gram-negative infection. The observed series of events, whereby a foreign molecule (i.e., LPS) serves to both trigger and attenuate a programmed cellular stress response, suggests a novel homeostatic pathway for regulation of the acute phase response.

APOLIPOPROTEIN E AND MICROBIAL IMMUNITY

Although the capacity of triglyceride-rich lipoproteins to bind and neutralize LPS can be accurately predicted by the phospholipid content of the lipid particles, additional protein constituents also play an important role in the process. Apolipoprotein E (apoE), consistent with its ability to facilitate the clearance of triglyceride-rich lipoproteins by the liver, has been shown both to redirect LPS from Kupffer cells to hepatocytes and to protect against endotoxemia in rats [24]. ApoE–knockout mice are also more susceptible to LPS-induced lethality than are controls, despite elevated plasma lipid levels [72]. Similarly, when given intravenously, apoE has been shown to decrease LPS-induced morbidity and mortality in mice and has thus been identified to have anti-infective properties [73]. But, quite unexpectedly, our laboratory has recently discovered that infusion of apoE increased rather than decreased mortality after cecal ligation and puncture (CLP), an *in vivo* model of polymicrobial sepsis [74]. Interestingly, apoE has recently been implicated in the activation of Natural Killer T (NKT) cells by acting as a molecular chaperone for bacterial antigens, delivering them to antigen-presenting cells via LDLR to activate NKT cells by CD1d, a nonclassical class-I-like antigen-presenting molecule (Figure 3) [75]. Predominantly located in the liver, activated NKT cells can secrete large amounts of T_H1 and T_H2 cytokines and appear to serve as a bridge between innate and acquired immunity [76]. We therefore looked at NKT cell response in apoE-treated septic mice. ApoE treatment resulted in increased NKT number and proliferation, predominantly in the liver, with concomitant decreases in NKT cell number and proliferation in the periphery, implying hepatic trafficking. ApoE treatment also increased T_H1 response and hepatocellular injury. Taken together, these observations identify apoE as making a significant contribution to host defense against infection by regulating the processing of foreign lipid antigens during sepsis, and by activating NKT cells.

In contrast with earlier findings, these results argue against a protective role for apoE. A possible reason for the different findings is that we used serial injections of apoE in our CLP model of sepsis, whereas earlier studies used injection of LPS as a model for sepsis and demonstrated protection by pre-incubating LPS with apoE prior to injection. In an effort to determine whether the observed hyperactive inflammatory response induced by supraphysiologic concentrations of apoE was physiologically relevant, we have recently performed a series of experiments showing that hypomorphic apoE transgenic mice expressing 2-5% of wild type levels of apoE level are less susceptible to septic mortality than their induced, wild-type counterparts [unpublished]. These findings appear to validate the proinflammatory contribution that apoE makes in sepsis. It also indicates that a subphysiologic level of apoE is ideal in the face of sepsis. With all the findings to date, it appears that apoE may regulate a delicate counterbalance between systemic inflammation and pathogen clearance.

Expanding upon these findings is the first clinical study to examine the link between apoE polymorphism and sepsis risk in surgical patients [77]. The apoE gene codes for three main isoforms of the protein, designated apoE2, E3, and E4. Whereas the three isoforms only differ by a single amino acid substitution, they collectively constitute a range of LDLR binding affinities (E4>E3>>>E2). The prospective observational study looked at 343 patients with planned admission to the ICU following major elective noncardiac surgery. Carriers of the apoE3 allele experienced a lower incidence of severe sepsis after elective surgery than patients without this allele (p = 0.014, RR = 0.28). The protective effect remained significant after age, gender, and race were adjusted for. This study demonstrated the first clinical association between apolipoprotein E expression and sepsis. Although the mechanistic link between these findings and previous findings in animal models has yet to be established, all these studies point to a potential target in our efforts develop effective therapies for sepsis.

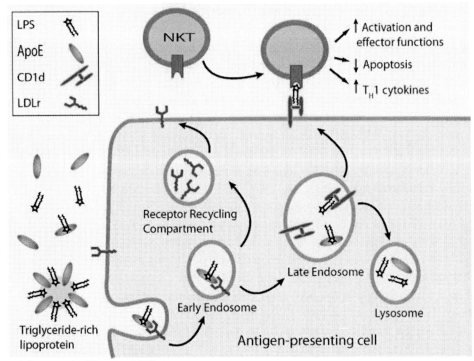

Adapted from van den Elzen *et al.* [75]

Figure 3. Proposed model of apolipoprotein E (apoE)-mediated lipid antigen presentation and NKT cell activation. Pathogenic microbial lipids (e.g. lipopolysaccharide, LPS) are delivered to antigen-presenting cells as part of a triglyceride-rich lipoprotein (i.e. chylomicrons and very low density lipoproteins) or bound to apoE. The lipid complex binds to the LDL receptor (LDLr), is internalized and while trafficked through the endosomal compartments, is processed and loaded onto CD1d for display on the cell surface where it activates CD1d-restricted NKT cells.

LIPID-BASED TREATMENT STRATEGIES

Considerable efforts have been expended to find novel therapeutic strategies to combat sepsis. Unfortunately, most of these strategies failed to improve patient survival when studied in large, multicenter clinical trials [78, 79]. Many of the pathways which were targeted, e.g., IL-1 and TNF-α, are part of an extensive redundant network that cannot be interrupted with an agent that blocks a single pathway. Lipoprotein involvement in endotoxin neutralization and uptake, in addition to apoE's role in activating innate immunity, provide potential targets for therapeutic intervention. These potential targets act further upstream in the inflammatory cascade than previous treatments and potentially exert a more global effect on decreasing inflammation.

Given that apoE hyperactivates the immune system presumably via LDLR-based antigen presentation, preventing this receptor-ligand interaction could decrease inflammation and septic mortality. Acting directly at the protein level, potential apoE antagonists include anti-apoE antibodies and soluble apoE receptors. ApoE siRNA and apoE anti-sense oligo-nucleotides could act further upstream to inhibit apoE transcription and translation. At the putative receptor level, high concentrations of noninflammatory apoE-mimetic peptides could outcompete native proinflammatory apoE for receptor binding sites. Similarly, an LDLR antagonist such as receptor-associated protein (RAP) could prevent apoE-LDLR interaction and the downstream cytokine response. In fact, LDLR-based therapy currently exists in statins, but the novel mechanism has only recently been alluded to.

HMG-CoA reductase inhibitors, or statins, in addition their cholesterol-lowering effects, also appear to have independent anti-inflammatory effects. Statin pretreatment improved survival in a murine sepsis model [80], and in a retrospective human study, statin therapy reduced mortality rates attributable to bacteremia [81]. Since statins increase LDLR expression, and LDL receptors internalize lipoproteins and endotoxin, it has been presumed that statins can enhance endotoxin clearance from the circulation and attenuate the septic response [82]. In addition to increased clearance of endotoxin, hepatocyte cytokine tolerance following internalization of lipoprotein-bound LPS can further minimize the proinflammatory effects of LPS.

CONCLUSION

LPS elicits dramatic changes in the host, including the increased synthesis and secretion of triglyceride-rich lipoproteins by the liver. This LPS-induced hyperlipoproteinemia, the "lipemia of sepsis," was customarily thought to represent the mobilization of lipid stores to fuel the host response to infection. But since lipoproteins can also bind and neutralize LPS, it has been postulated that triglyceride-rich lipoproteins are agents of an innate, non-adaptive host immune response. Interestingly, the LPS-lipoprotein binding process entails the insertion of the lipophilic lipid A domain of endotoxin into the phospholipid surface of the accepting lipoprotein and is facilitated by CD14 and LBP, itself an acute phase protein. Once inserted, the ability of the lipid A moiety to stimulate LPS-responsive cells and tissues is greatly reduced. Furthermore, the catabolism of LPS subsequently mirrors that of the lipoprotein with which it is associated. When LPS is bound to a triglyceride-rich lipoprotein it is rapidly cleared from the circulation by hepatocytes. Subsequently, the internalized lipoprotein-LPS complex exerts an anti-inflammatory effect, attenuating the cytokine-mediated activation of NF-κB, and thus serves to regulate the acute phase response. Several studies have shown that elevated plasma lipoprotein levels are protective against LPS-mediated toxicity in vertebrates. On the basis of recent studies, apolipoprotein E appears to be a key mediator of immunoregulation likely due to selective Natural Killer T cell activation and T_H1 cytokine secretion. Ultimately, a better understanding of how triglyceride-rich lipoproteins and their components modulate the body's response to LPS could yield novel biological insights with important clinical implications.

REFERENCES

[1]   Banerjee, S; Bhaduri, JN. Serum protein-bound carbohydrates and lipids in cholera. Proc Soc Exp Biol Med, 1959. 101(2), 340-1.

[2]   Gallin, JI; Kaye, D; O'Leary, WM. Serum lipids in infection. N Engl J Med, 1969. 281(20), 1081-6.

[3]   Samra, JS; Summers, LK; Frayn, KN. Sepsis and fat metabolism. Br J Surg, 1996.
        83(9), 1186-96.

[4]   Tripp, RJ; Tabares, A; Wang, H; Lanza-Jacoby, S. Altered hepatic production of
        apolipoproteins B and E in the fasted septic rat: factors in the development of
        hypertriglyceridemia. J Surg Res, 1993. 55(5), 465-72.

[5]   Wolfe, RR; Shaw, JH; Durkot, MJ. Effect of sepsis on VLDL kinetics: responses in
        basal state and during glucose infusion. Am J Physiol, 1985. 248(6 Pt 1), E732-40.

[6]   Feingold, KR; Marshall, M; Gulli, R; Moser, AH; Grunfeld, C. Effect of endotoxin and
        cytokines on lipoprotein lipase activity in mice. Arterioscler Thromb, 1994. 14(11),
        1866-72.

[7]   Feingold, KR; Serio, MK; Adi, S; Moser, AH; Grunfeld, C. Tumor necrosis factor
        stimulates hepatic lipid synthesis and secretion. Endocrinology, 1989. 124(5), 2336-42.

[8]   Feingold, KR; Soued, M; Staprans, I; Gavin, LA; Donahue, ME; Huang, BJ; Moser,
        AH; Gulli, R; Grunfeld, C. Effect of tumor necrosis factor (TNF) on lipid metabolism
        in the diabetic rat. Evidence that inhibition of adipose tissue lipoprotein lipase activity
        is not required for TNF-induced hyperlipidemia. J Clin Invest, 1989. 83(4), 1116-21.

[9]   Starnes, HF; Jr; Warren, RS; Jeevanandam, M; Gabrilove, JL; Larchian, W; Oettgen,
        HF; Brennan, MF. Tumor necrosis factor and the acute metabolic response to tissue
        injury in man. J Clin Invest, 1988. 82(4), 1321-5.

[10]   Nonogaki, K; Moser, AH; Feingold, KR; Grunfeld, C. Alpha-adrenergic receptors
        mediate the hypertriglyceridemia induced by endotoxin, but not tumor necrosis factor,
        in rats. Endocrinology, 1994. 135(6), 2644-50.

[11]   Lanza-Jacoby, S; Phetteplace, H; Sedkova, N; Knee, G. Sequential alterations in tissue
        lipoprotein lipase, triglyceride secretion rates, and serum tumor necrosis factor alpha
        during Escherichia coli bacteremic sepsis in relation to the development of
        hypertriglyceridemia. Shock, 1998. 9(1), 46-51.

[12]   Scholl, RA; Lang, CH; Bagby, GJ. Hypertriglyceridemia and its relation to tissue
        lipoprotein lipase activity in endotoxemic, Escherichia coli bacteremic, and
        polymicrobial septic rats. J Surg Res, 1984. 37(5), 394-401.

[13]   Feingold, KR; Staprans, I; Memon, RA; Moser, AH; Shigenaga, JK; Doerrler, W;
        Dinarello, CA; Grunfeld, C. Endotoxin rapidly induces changes in lipid metabolism that
        produce hypertriglyceridemia: low doses stimulate hepatic triglyceride production
        while high doses inhibit clearance. J Lipid Res, 1992. 33(12), 1765-76.

[14]   Eichbaum, EB; Harris, HW; Kane, JP; Rapp, JH. Chylomicrons can inhibit endotoxin
        activity in vitro. J Surg Res, 1991. 51(5), 413-6.

[15]   Harris, HW; Eichbaum, EB; Kane, JP; Rapp, JH. Detection of endotoxin in triglyceride-
        rich lipoproteins in vitro. J Lab Clin Med, 1991. 118(2), 186-93.

[16]   Ulevitch, RJ; Johnston, AR. The modification of biophysical and endotoxic properties
        of bacterial lipopolysaccharides by serum. J Clin Invest, 1978. 62(6), 1313-24.

[17]   Ulevitch, RJ; Johnston, AR. Weinstein, DB. New function for high density lipoproteins.
        Their participation in intravascular reactions of bacterial lipopolysaccharides. J Clin
        Invest, 1979. 64(5), 1516-24.

[18]   Ulevitch, RJ; Johnston, AR; Weinstein, DB. New function for high density lipoproteins.
        Isolation and characterization of a bacterial lipopolysaccharide-high density lipoprotein
        complex formed in rabbit plasma. J Clin Invest, 1981. 67(3), 827-37.

[19] Van Lenten, BJ; Fogelman, AM; Haberland, ME; Edwards, PA. The role of lipoproteins and receptor-mediated endocytosis in the transport of bacterial lipopolysaccharide. Proc Natl Acad Sci U S A, 1986. 83(8), 2704-8.

[20] Navab, M; Hough, GP; Van Lenten, BJ; Berliner, JA; Fogelman, AM. Low density lipoproteins transfer bacterial lipopolysaccharides across endothelial monolayers in a biologically active form. J Clin Invest, 1988. 81(2), 601-5.

[21] Harris, HW; Grunfeld, C; Feingold, KR; Rapp, JH. Human very low density lipoproteins and chylomicrons can protect against endotoxin-induced death in mice. J Clin Invest, 1990. 86(3), 696-702.

[22] Cue, JI; DiPiro, JT; Brunner, LJ; Doran, JE; Blankenship, ME; Mansberger, AR; Hawkins, ML. Reconstituted high density lipoprotein inhibits physiologic and tumor necrosis factor alpha responses to lipopolysaccharide in rabbits. Arch Surg, 1994. 129(2), 193-7.

[23] Parker, TS; Levine, DM; Chang, JC; Laxer, J; Coffin, CC; Rubin, AL. Reconstituted high-density lipoprotein neutralizes gram-negative bacterial lipopolysaccharides in human whole blood. Infect Immun, 1995. 63(1), 253-8.

[24] Rensen, PC; Oosten, M; Bilt, E; Eck, M; Kuiper, J; Berkel, TJ. Human recombinant apolipoprotein E redirects lipopolysaccharide from Kupffer cells to liver parenchymal cells in rats In vivo. J Clin Invest, 1997. 99(10), 2438-45.

[25] Wright, SD; Ramos, RA; Tobias, PS; Ulevitch, RJ; Mathison, JC. CD14, a receptor for complexes of lipopolysaccharide (LPS) and LPS binding protein. Science, 1990. 249(4975), 1431-3.

[26] Landmann, R; Muller, B; Zimmerli, W. CD14, new aspects of ligand and signal diversity. Microbes Infect, 2000. 2(3), 295-304.

[27] Schumann, RR; Zweigner, J. A novel acute-phase marker: lipopolysaccharide binding protein (LBP). Clin Chem Lab Med, 1999. 37(3), 271-4.

[28] Schutt, C. Fighting infection: the role of lipopolysaccharide binding proteins CD14 and LBP. Pathobiology, 1999. 67(5-6), 227-9.

[29] Van Voorhis, WC; Steinman, RM; Hair, LS; Luban, J; Witmer, MD; Koide, S; Cohn, ZA. Specific antimononuclear phagocyte monoclonal antibodies. Application to the purification of dendritic cells and the tissue localization of macrophages. J Exp Med, 1983. 158(1), 126-45.

[30] Haziot, A; Chen, S; Ferrero, E; Low, MG; Silber, R; Goyert, SM. The monocyte differentiation antigen, CD14, is anchored to the cell membrane by a phosphatidylinositol linkage. J Immunol, 1988. 141(2), 547-52.

[31] Lynn, WA; Liu, Y; Golenbock, DT. Neither CD14 nor serum is absolutely necessary for activation of mononuclear phagocytes by bacterial lipopolysaccharide. Infect Immun, 1993. 61(10), 4452-61.

[32] Triantafilou, M; Triantafilou, K; Fernandez, N. Rough and smooth forms of fluorescein-labelled bacterial endotoxin exhibit CD14/LBP dependent and independent binding that is influencedby endotoxin concentration. Eur J Biochem, 2000. 267(8), 2218-26.

[33] Troelstra, A; Antal-Szalmas, P; de Graaf-Miltenburg, LA; Weersink, AJ; Verhoef, J; Van Kessel, KP; Van Strijp, JA. Saturable CD14-dependent binding of fluorescein-labeled lipopolysaccharide to human monocytes. Infect Immun, 1997. 65(6), 2272-7.

[34] Maliszewski, CR; Ball, ED; Graziano, RF; Fanger, MW. Isolation and characterization of My23, a myeloid cell-derived antigen reactive with the monoclonal antibody AML-2-23. J Immunol, 1985. 135(3), 1929-36.

[35] Bazil, V; Horejsi, V; Baudys, M; Kristofova, H; Strominger, JL; Kostka, W; Hilgert, I. Biochemical characterization of a soluble form of the 53-kDa monocyte surface antigen. Eur J Immunol, 1986. 16(12), 1583-9.

[36] Frey, EA; Miller, DS; Jahr, TG; Sundan, A; Bazil, V; Espevik, T; Finlay, BB; Wright, SD. Soluble CD14 participates in the response of cells to lipopolysaccharide. J Exp Med, 1992. 176(6), 1665-71.

[37] Pugin, J; Schurer-Maly, CC; Leturcq, D; Moriarty, A; Ulevitch, RJ; Tobias, PS. Lipopolysaccharide activation of human endothelial and epithelial cells is mediated by lipopolysaccharide-binding protein and soluble CD14. Proc Natl Acad Sci U S A, 1993. 90(7), 2744-8.

[38] Hailman, E; Lichenstein, HS; Wurfel, MM; Miller, DS; Johnson, DA; Kelley, M; Busse, LA; Zukowski, MM; Wright, SD. Lipopolysaccharide (LPS)-binding protein accelerates the binding of LPS to CD14. J Exp Med, 1994. 179(1), 269-77.

[39] Haziot, A; Rong, GW; Silver, J; Goyert, SM. Recombinant soluble CD14 mediates the activation of endothelial cells by lipopolysaccharide. J Immunol, 1993. 151(3), 1500-7.

[40] Read, MA; Cordle, SR; Veach, RA; Carlisle, CD; Hawiger, J. Cell-free pool of CD14 mediates activation of transcription factor NF-kappa B by lipopolysaccharide in human endothelial cells. Proc Natl Acad Sci U S A, 1993. 90(21), 9887-91.

[41] Ulevitch, RJ; Tobias, PS. Receptor-dependent mechanisms of cell stimulation by bacterial endotoxin. Annu Rev Immunol, 1995. 13, 437-57.

[42] Beamer, LJ; Carroll, SF; Eisenberg, D. Crystal structure of human BPI and two bound phospholipids at 2.4 angstrom resolution. Science, 1997. 276(5320), 1861-4.

[43] Elsbach, P. The bactericidal/permeability-increasing protein (BPI) in antibacterial host defense. J Leukoc Biol, 1998. 64(1), 14-8.

[44] Tall, A; Plasma lipid transfer proteins. Annu Rev Biochem, 1995. 64, 235-57.

[45] Wurfel, MM; Wright, SD. Lipopolysaccharide-binding protein and soluble CD14 transfer lipopolysaccharide to phospholipid bilayers: preferential interaction with particular classes of lipid. J Immunol, 1997. 158(8), 3925-34.

[46] Yu, B; Wright, SD. Catalytic properties of lipopolysaccharide (LPS) binding protein. Transfer of LPS to soluble CD14. J Biol Chem, 1996. 271(8), 4100-5.

[47] Vesy, CJ; Kitchens, RL; Wolfbauer, G; Albers, JJ; Munford, RS. Lipopolysaccharide-binding protein and phospholipid transfer protein release lipopolysaccharides from gram-negative bacterial membranes. Infect Immun, 2000. 68(5), 2410-7.

[48] Kitchens, RL; Wolfbauer, G; Albers, JJ; Munford, RS. Plasma lipoproteins promote the release of bacterial lipopolysaccharide from the monocyte cell surface. J Biol Chem, 1999. 274(48), 34116-22.

[49] Netea, MG; Demacker, PN; Kullberg, BJ; Jacobs, LE; Verver-Jansen, TJ; Boerman, OC; Stalenhoef, AF. Van der Meer, JW. Bacterial lipopolysaccharide binds and stimulates cytokine-producing cells before neutralization by endogenous lipoproteins can occur. Cytokine, 1998. 10(10), 766-72.

[50] Harris, HW; Johnson, JA; Wigmore, SJ. Endogenous lipoproteins impact the response to endotoxin in humans. Crit Care Med, 2002. 30(1), 23-31.

[51]   Feingold, KR; Funk, JL; Moser, AH; Shigenaga, JK; Rapp, JH; Grunfeld, C. Role for circulating lipoproteins in protection from endotoxin toxicity. Infect Immun, 1995. 63(5), 2041-6.

[52]   Read, TE; Grunfeld, C; Kumwenda, Z; Calhoun, MC; Kane, JP; Feingold, KR; Rapp, JH. Triglyceride-rich lipoproteins improve survival when given after endotoxin in rats. Surgery, 1995. 117(1), 62-7.

[53]   Casas, AT; Hubsch, AP; Doran, JE. Effects of reconstituted high-density lipoprotein in persistent gram-negative bacteremia. Am Surg, 1996. 62(5), 350-5.

[54]   Casas, AT; Hubsch, AP; Rogers, BC; Doran, JE. Reconstituted high-density lipoprotein reduces LPS-stimulated TNF alpha. J Surg Res, 1995. 59(5), 544-52.

[55]   Hubsch, AP; Powell, FS; Lerch, PG; Doran, JE. A reconstituted, apolipoprotein A-I containing lipoprotein reduces tumor necrosis factor release and attenuates shock in endotoxemic rabbits. Circ Shock, 1993. 40(1), 14-23.

[56]   Pajkrt, D; Doran, JE; Koster, F; Lerch, PG; Arnet, B; van der Poll, T; ten Cate, JW; van Deventer, SJ. Antiinflammatory effects of reconstituted high-density lipoprotein during human endotoxemia. J Exp Med, 1996. 184(5), 1601-8.

[57]   Levine, DM; Parker, TS; Donnelly, TM; Walsh, A; Rubin, AL. In vivo protection against endotoxin by plasma high density lipoprotein. Proc Natl Acad Sci U S A, 1993. 90(24), 12040-4.

[58]   Harris, HW; Rockey, DC; Young, DM; Welch, WJ. Diet-induced protection against lipopolysaccharide includes increased hepatic NO production. J Surg Res, 1999. 82(2), 339-45.

[59]   van der Poll, T; Braxton, CC; Coyle, SM; Boermeester, MA; Wang, JC; Jansen, PM; Montegut, WJ; Calvano, SE; Hack, CE; Lowry, SF. Effect of hypertriglyceridemia on endotoxin responsiveness in humans. Infect Immun, 1995. 63(9), 3396-400.

[60]   Abe, M; Kawano, M; Tashiro, T; Yamamori, H; Takagi, K; Morishima, Y; Shirai, K; Saitou, Y; Nakajima, N. Catabolism of lipoprotein-X induced by infusion of 10% fat emulsion. Nutrition, 1997. 13(5), 417-21.

[61]   Ferezou, J; Nguyen, TL; Leray, C; Hajri, T; Frey, A; Cabaret, Y; Courtieu, J; Lutton, C; Bach, AC. Lipid composition and structure of commercial parenteral emulsions. Biochim Biophys Acta, 1994. 1213(2), 149-58.

[62]   Hajri, T; Ferezou, J; Lutton, C. Effects of intravenous infusions of commercial fat emulsions (Intralipid 10 or 20%) on rat plasma lipoproteins: phospholipids in excess are the main precursors of lipoprotein-X-like particles. Biochim Biophys Acta, 1990. 1047(2), 121-30.

[63]   Hultin, M; Carneheim, C; Rosenqvist, K; Olivecrona, T. Intravenous lipid emulsions: removal mechanisms as compared to chylomicrons. J Lipid Res, 1995. 36(10), 2174-84.

[64]   Karpe, F; Hultin, M. Endogenous triglyceride-rich lipoproteins accumulate in rat plasma when competing with a chylomicron-like triglyceride emulsion for a common lipolytic pathway. J Lipid Res, 1995. 36(7), 1557-66.

[65]   Tashiro, T; Mashima, Y; Yamamori, H; Sanada, M; Nishizawa, M. Okui. K. Intravenous intralipid 10% vs. 20%, hyperlipidemia, and increase in lipoprotein X in humans. Nutrition, 1992. 8(3), 155-60.

[66]   Harris, HW; Grunfeld, C; Feingold, KR; Read, TE; Kane, JP; Jones, AL; Eichbaum, EB; Bland, GF; Rapp, JH. Chylomicrons alter the fate of endotoxin, decreasing tumor necrosis factor release and preventing death. J Clin Invest, 1993. 91(3), 1028-34.

[67] Harris, HW; Rockey, DC; Chau, P. Chylomicrons alter the hepatic distribution and cellular response to endotoxin in rats. Hepatology, 1998. 27(5), 1341-8.

[68] Flegel, WA; Baumstark, MW; Weinstock, C; Berg, A; Northoff, H. Prevention of endotoxin-induced monokine release by human low- and high-density lipoproteins and by apolipoprotein A-I. Infect Immun, 1993. 61(12), 5140-6.

[69] Flegel, WA; Wolpl, A; Mannel, DN; Northoff, H. Inhibition of endotoxin-induced activation of human monocytes by human lipoproteins. Infect Immun, 1989. 57(7), 2237-45.

[70] Weinstock, C; Ullrich, H; Hohe, R; Berg, A; Baumstark, MW; Frey, I; Northoff, H; Flegel, WA. Low density lipoproteins inhibit endotoxin activation of monocytes. Arterioscler Thromb, 1992. 12(3), 341-7.

[71] Kumwenda, ZL; Wong, CB; Johnson, JA; Gosnell, JE; Welch, WJ; Harris, HW. Chylomicron-bound endotoxin selectively inhibits NF-kappaB activation in rat hepatocytes. Shock, 2002. 18(2), 182-8.

[72] de Bont, N; Netea, MG; Demacker, PN; Verschueren, I; Kullberg, BJ; van Dijk, KW; van der Meer, JW; Stalenhoef, AF. Apolipoprotein E knock-out mice are highly susceptible to endotoxemia and Klebsiella pneumoniae infection. J Lipid Res, 1999. 40(4), 680-5.

[73] Roselaar, SE; Daugherty, A. Apolipoprotein E-deficient mice have impaired innate immune responses to Listeria monocytogenes in vivo. J Lipid Res, 1998. 39(9), 1740-3.

[74] Kattan, OM; Kasravi, FB; Elford, EL; Schell, MT; Harris, HW. Apolipoprotein E-mediated immune regulation in sepsis. J Immunol, 2008. 181(2), 1399-408.

[75] van den Elzen, P; Garg, S; Leon, L; Brigl, M; Leadbetter, EA; Gumperz, JE; Dascher, CC; Cheng, TY; Sacks, FM; Illarionov, PA; Besra, GS; Kent, SC; Moody, DB; Brenner, MB. Apolipoprotein-mediated pathways of lipid antigen presentation. Nature, 2005. 437(7060), 906-10.

[76] Taniguchi, M; Seino, K; Nakayama, T. The NKT cell system: bridging innate and acquired immunity. Nat Immunol, 2003. 4(12), 1164-5.

[77] Moretti, EW; Morris, RW; Podgoreanu, M; Schwinn, DA; Newman, MF; Bennett, E; Moulin, VG; Mba, UU; Laskowitz, DT. APOE polymorphism is associated with risk of severe sepsis in surgical patients. Crit Care Med, 2005. 33(11), 2521-6.

[78] Bochud, PY; Calandra, T. Pathogenesis of sepsis: new concepts and implications for future treatment. BMJ, 2003. 326(7383), 262-6.

[79] Riedemann, NC; Guo, RF; Ward, PA. Novel strategies for the treatment of sepsis. Nat Med, 2003. 9(5), 517-24.

[80] Merx, MW; Liehn, EA; Janssens, U; Lutticken, R; Schrader, J; Hanrath, P; Weber, C. HMG-CoA reductase inhibitor simvastatin profoundly improves survival in a murine model of sepsis. Circulation, 2004. 109(21), 2560-5.

[81] Liappis, AP; Kan, VL; Rochester, CG; Simon, G.L. The effect of statins on mortality in patients with bacteremia. Clin Infect Dis, 2001. 33(8), 1352-7.

[82] Spitzer, AL; Harris, HW. Statins attenuate sepsis. Surgery, 2006. 139(3), 283-7.

In: Sepsis: Symptoms, Diagnosis and Treatment
Editor: Joseph R. Brown, pp. 93-105

ISBN: 978-1-60876-609-3
© 2010 Nova Science Publishers, Inc.

Chapter 5

IMPROVEMENT OF EARLY RECOGNITION AND TREATMENT OF PATIENTS WITH SEPSIS: AREAS THAT NEED TO BE EXPLORED

Mirjam Tromp[1], Chantal P. Bleeker-Rovers[1] and Peter Pickkers[2]

[1]Department of Internal Medicine, [2]Department of Intensive Care
Nijmegen Institute for Infection, Inflammation, and Immunity (N4i),
Radboud University Nijmegen Medical Centre, The Netherlands

ABSTRACT

In 2004, the Surviving Sepsis Campaign (SSC) was launched to improve the recognition, diagnosis, management, and treatment of sepsis. From that moment on a vast amount of articles concerning the early recognition and treatment of patients with sepsis and different tools to measure and improve the quality of care for patients with sepsis have been published. Although the SSC supplies tools to measure and improve the quality of care for patients with sepsis, no recommendations concerning the role of the nurses are given and effective implementation remains troublesome.

This chapter will mainly focus on the fact that early recognition and treatment of septic patients admitted to the ED can significantly improve after introduction of a predominantly nurse-driven sepsis registration protocol and education and feedback regarding its performance. An overview of the existing literature concerning general implementation techniques, focusing on different steps in the implementation process, is given. Apart from this overview, the effects of a predominantly nurse-driven prospective before-and-after intervention study at the emergency department are described. Compared to previous performed studies, this described new implementation technique was very successful. After the performance of the entire implementation program, four out of six recommendations and the compliance with the bundle of six recommendations improved significantly. It was demonstrated that four patient characteristics influenced the overall compliance rate to the sepsis protocol: patients' age, CRP result, ICU admission, and the final diagnosis.

In addition, following an educational intervention about sepsis, it was possible to improve residents' knowledge about sepsis definitions, and diagnosis and treatment of sepsis. Apart from the short-term effects, the improved test results were sustained after 4-6 months.

INTRODUCTION

Approximately 2% of all hospitalized patients are diagnosed with severe sepsis or septic shock. Intensive care and the long recovery period for patients with sepsis are accompanied with high costs. Also, mortality is very high: 30-40% in severe sepsis and 40-50% in septic shock [1-3]. Rapid diagnosis and management of sepsis is critical for successful treatment. Although the Surviving Sepsis Campaign (SSC) supplies tools to measure and improve the quality of care for patients with sepsis, no recommendations concerning the role of nurses are provided and effective implementation remains troublesome.

Sepsis Definitions

Standardization of terminology is necessary to eliminate confusion in communication for both clinicians and researchers. Several editorials and position papers have attempted to provide a framework for standardization and simplification of the sepsis terminology [4-7]. In 1992, the ACCP/SCCM Consensus Conference Committee offered recommendations for the standardization of the sepsis terminology [8].

Sepsis: the systemic response to (strongly suspected or proven) infection, manifested by two or more of the following conditions as a result of infection: (1) temperature >38°C or <36°C; (2) heart rate >90 beats per minute; (3) respiratory rate >20 breaths per minute or $PaCO_2$ <32 mmHg; and (4) white blood cell count >12,000/mm^3, <4,000/mm^3, or >10% immature (band) forms.

Severe sepsis: sepsis associated with organ dysfunction, hypo-perfusion, or hypotension. Hypoperfusion and perfusion abnormalities may include, but are not limited to, lactic acidosis, oliguria, and an acute alteration in mental status.

Septic shock: sepsis with hypotension despite adequate fluid resuscitation along with the presence of perfusion abnormalities that may include, but are not limited to, lactic acidosis, oliguria, and an acute alteration in mental status. Patients who are receiving inotropic or vasopressor agents may not be hypotensive at the time perfusion abnormalities are measured, but are also considered as suffering from septic shock.

THE SURVIVING SEPSIS CAMPAIGN AT THE EMERGENCY DEPARTMENT

To improve rapid diagnosis and management of sepsis, the SSC provides helpful tools and some implementation techniques to measure and improve the quality of care for patients with sepsis, especially for patients in the intensive care unit. The most important recommendations are summarized in a '6 hour' and '24 hour' bundle: the resuscitation bundle and the management bundle [1-3;9-11].

The majority of septic patients present themselves at the emergency department (ED) [12].

It is becoming increasingly clear that time is an important factor not only in trauma patients and patients suffering from myocardial infarction or a cerebral vascular accident, but also in patients with severe sepsis or septic shock since they have a better chance of survival if sepsis is recognized and treated adequately at an earlier stage [13]. Research shows that in a hypotensive septic patient, every hour that the first administration of adequate antimicrobial therapy is delayed, is associated with an increase in mortality of 8% [14]. Due to the high mortality-rate for patients with severe sepsis and septic shock at the ED [15], the ED is an important location for early recognition and treatment of sepsis. For diagnosis and treatment of sepsis at the ED, recommendations from the resuscitation bundle are important. These recommendations must be accomplished within the first 6 hours after presentation at the ED.

Recommendations from the resuscitation bundle:

1. Measure serum lactate;
2. Obtain blood cultures prior to antibiotic administration;
3. Administer broad-spectrum antibiotic within 3 hours of ED admission and within 1 hour of non-ED admission;
4. In the event of hypotension and/or serum lactate >4 mmol/L:
    (a) Deliver an initial minimum of 20 ml/kg of crystalloid or an equivalent
    (b) Apply vasopressors for hypotension not responding to initial fluid resuscitation to maintain mean arterial pressure (MAP) >65 mm Hg;
5. In the event of persistent hypotension despite fluid resuscitation (septic shock) and/or lactate >4 mmol/L:
    (a) Achieve a central venous pressure (CVP) of ≥ 8 mm Hg
    (b) Achieve a central venous oxygen saturation (ScvO2) $\geq 70\%$ or mixed venous oxygen saturation (SvO2) $\geq 65\%$.

Although these recommendations focus on patients with severe sepsis or septic shock, all septic patients need to be screened to recognize the most affected. Thus, these recommendations should be applied to all septic patients. The first step to reduce the mortality in severe sepsis and septic shock is to prevent the progression of sepsis to severe sepsis and septic shock [16]. It is to be expected that this can be reached by the early recognition and treatment of patients with sepsis. However, most studies about implementation of the resuscitation bundle specifically focus on patients with severe sepsis and septic shock [17-21].

The Role of Nurses at The Emergency Department

As nurses are often the first to see and triage a patient, their position in the current organization structure should be exploited to a greater extent. So far, no specific attention to the screening role of nurses is given [9-11]. It is important to educate ED nurses about the symptoms of sepsis and the performance of the actions from the resuscitation bundle. In a study that was carried out to assess nurses' knowledge of sepsis, it was shown that identification of septic patients is a problem, e.g., only approximately 20% of the respondents thought that a temperature <36°C or a low white cell count could be signs of sepsis [22].

IMPLEMENTATION OF A NURSE-DRIVEN SEPSIS PROTOCOL

A sepsis protocol can be successfully implemented in the ED in five steps:

1. Determination of the Problem

Several studies have shown that 30-40% of patients do not receive care according to the present scientific evidence and 20-25% of the care provided is not needed or potentially harmful [23;24]. To achieve an improvement in quality of care in the ED, a random check of patients that have been admitted to the ED with (severe) sepsis should be performed. Results obtained in a retrospective analysis should include quality of diagnostics and time to treatment.

2. Choosing an Aim of the Project That is Borne by the Organization

A major determinant for a successful project includes choosing an aim that is borne by the whole organization. If possible, the project should be incorporated in existing quality initiatives in the hospital. Using the results obtained in the retrospective analysis of patients with severe sepsis that were admitted to the ED, aims can be formulated to improve the diagnostics and treatment of these patients.
Examples:

- To improve the registration of all septic patients presenting at the ED facilitating the possibility to acquire information about the quality of care for patients with (severe) sepsis/septic shock admitted to the ED.
- To formulate possible ways to improve care for these patients.
- To improve the diagnostic and therapeutic process for patients with severe sepsis/septic shock on the ED by implementation of the SSC guidelines.

3. The Development of a Nurse-Driven Sepsis Protocol

A sepsis protocol for the ED should be developed by a multidisciplinary team including an intensive care specialist, internal medicine physicians, a surgeon, a medical microbiologist, a clinical pharmacist, ED nurses, and a nurse practitioner. All persons involved have to be familiar with the hospital organization, organization at the ED, and the professionals working at the ED. They have to combine evidence from the literature about strategies for the development of a protocol [25-27] and the sepsis guidelines with expert opinion. To improve the early identification of septic patients at the ED, a sepsis screening list should be developed (figure 1) to support the nurses at the ED in better recognition of sepsis in patients with a probable infection. In addition, a checklist/registration form with recommendations for nurses and physicians at the ED should be introduced (figure 2).

The most important changes for the nurses in the ED following the initiation of the sepsis protocol include:

- The role of the nurses during the triage of patients with suspicion of sepsis will be extended;
- Timing of essential procedures must be registered;
- The role of the nurses of the ED during the initiation of the diagnostics will be extended;
- It will be clearly described when an intensive care specialist needs to be consulted in severely ill patients;
- Antibiotics should be administered within 3 hours, but preferably within 1 hour after admission to the ED.

The development of the sepsis protocol and determination of essential parts of the diagnostic and therapeutic process form the first step in the implementation of the changes that need to be achieved. This process clarifies which part of the care for these patients is important and who is responsible.

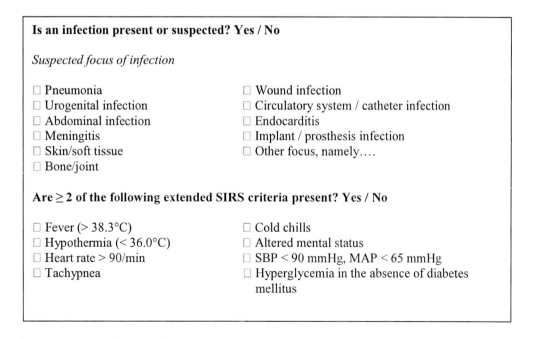

Is an infection present or suspected? Yes / No

Suspected focus of infection

☐ Pneumonia   ☐ Wound infection
☐ Urogenital infection   ☐ Circulatory system / catheter infection
☐ Abdominal infection   ☐ Endocarditis
☐ Meningitis   ☐ Implant / prosthesis infection
☐ Skin/soft tissue   ☐ Other focus, namely….
☐ Bone/joint

Are ≥ 2 of the following extended SIRS criteria present? Yes / No

☐ Fever (> 38.3°C)   ☐ Cold chills
☐ Hypothermia (< 36.0°C)   ☐ Altered mental status
☐ Heart rate > 90/min   ☐ SBP < 90 mmHg, MAP < 65 mmHg
☐ Tachypnea   ☐ Hyperglycemia in the absence of diabetes
                                  mellitus

Figure 1. Screening list for patients with (suspicion of) sepsis

Diagnostics	Initials	Time
Take blood samples (within 1 hour after admission to the ED) □ *Lactate, glucose, sodium, potassium, C-reactive protein, urea, creatinine, ASAT, ALAT, LD, alkaline phosphatase, bilirubin, hemoglobin, hematocrit, thrombocyte count , leukocyte count, differentiation, APTT, INR* □ *Take 2 blood cultures (before start antibiotics)*		
Standard diagnostics (within 1 hour after admission at the ED) □ *ECG* □ *Chest X-ray* □ *Urinalysis and urine culture*		
Depending on the focus of infection: take supplementary cultures before administration of antibiotics (within 1 hour after admission to the ED) □ *Sputum culture ....* □ *Feces culture ....* □ *Cerebrospinal fluid ....* □ *Other; ....*		
Treatment		

Administration of antibiotics (within 3 hours after admission to the ED)
Antibiotics administered?
□ *Yes*   *Name + doses of antibiotic treatment:*
       ..
       ..
□ *No: reason;* *..*		

In case of serum lactate > 4.0 mmol/L or hypotension: volume resuscitation 20 ml/kg crystalloid in max. 30 minutes *Was volume resuscitation needed?* □ *Yes; ....* □ *No*		
Hospitalization or discharge		

Figure 2. Checklist/registration form for patients with (suspicion of) sepsis

4. A Literature Overview on Implementation Strategies

For the implementation of a sepsis protocol, changes on the level of the organization, the department, a treatment team, and the individual care giver are needed [25]. Since these levels are usually related to each other, a team approach, in which different disciplines are represented, is necessary. To be successful in this change of care, the participants involved should be able to rely on their team in combination with the recognition of the need for the change. This way changes with a proven value can obtain a structural place in the daily routine of the ED nurses, in addition to the functioning of the organization as a whole.

Several models for implementation are known [28;29]. During the implementation of a sepsis protocol in the ED it is possible to use the model described by Grol &Wensing [25;26;30;31], in which the following 4 steps are recognized.

I.   Assess the possibilities for implementation of change: determine the chance of a successful implementation;
    (a) Create support for the new protocol.

(b) Determine relevant characteristics of the change.

(c) Adjust the change according to the wishes of the people that will use the protocol.

II. Diagnose the current situation: identify factors that influence implementation;

(a) Determine aims and goals of the personnel who will use the protocol.

(b) Clarify the current process. Determine barriers to and factors that promote changes. Determine subgroups in the personnel who will use the protocol.

III. Strategy of implementation: create a program for implementation;

(a) Choose one or more interventions.

(b) Create a plan to carry out the implementation. Determine how the change will be sustained.

IV. Evaluation: determine the course and effect of implementation and adjust the implementation plan if necessary;

(a) Evaluate the effects.

(b) Evaluate the course of the implementation.

(c) Evaluate the costs in relation to its effects.

It is important to realize that the above described steps are not a linear process but should be viewed as a cyclic process. To follow these steps may be considered as over the top and not necessary in daily practice, however, investing in this part of the implementation process is essential for successful implementation.

Implementation of a protocol is difficult and is seldom achieved without problems. Several barriers for a successful implementation of a protocol can be present [32-34]. This can start at the initiative to develop the protocol including lack of time or lack of the feeling of urgency to develop a protocol. During the implementation individual factors can be experienced as barriers by the members of the target group: employees are not aware of the guideline or protocol, they are not aware of the exact content of the protocol, they do not agree with the protocol, or they have no confidence in their own professionalism. Also, when there is a lack of confidence that the protocol will lead to better results or there is a lack of motivation to change, a successful implementation will be hampered [34]. In addition, social factors within teams and networks of care givers and within the organization related to the department or hospital influence the success of implementation.

Use of the SSC tools may be hindered by a variety of barriers to guideline adherence: lack of familiarity, lack of awareness, lack of agreement, lack of outcome expectancy, lack of self-efficacy, lack of motivation/inertia of previous practice, and external barriers [32]. Previous studies have demonstrated that an important reason for not following the SSC guidelines is that the identification of patients with sepsis can be difficult, resulting in treatment delay [22;33]. Only approximately 30% of physicians correctly identified Systemic Inflammatory Response Syndrome (SIRS) criteria [35]. Even after an active implementation of a sepsis teaching program, only 48% and 67% of the training-grade doctors respectively could define severe sepsis and septic shock [36]. Another reason for not following the SSC guidelines was shown to be the lack of knowledge about the management of patients with sepsis. Therefore, extensive knowledge about sepsis is an important condition for early identification and management of patients with sepsis.

To achieve a successful implementation, a strategic method in which it is important to determine and deal with different barriers is very important. The ultimate target should be that the change is maintained in daily practice. Therefore, repeated feedback about the results and effects is essential.

5. Implementation of the Protocol in Daily Practice

Based on the previously described theory [25;26;30;31], a summarized description of a guideline or protocol implementation in practice will be represented.

I. Assess the possibilities to implement the proposed change of practice

To get an impression of the medical support for implementation of a sepsis protocol in the ED, the plans and content of the protocol have to be discussed with the ED management and -nurses. Also, suggestions for improvement of the documents have to be discussed. In this way, the final sepsis protocol will fit the wishes and possibilities of the sepsis protocol users best.

II. Diagnose the current situation

Through the performance of a retrospective random check it is possible to gain an insight into the current care for patients with (severe) sepsis/septic shock in the ED. Differences between daily practice and sepsis protocol based theory regarding diagnostics and treatment of patients with sepsis can be determined. The persons involved in the implementation of the sepsis protocol have to be identified (mainly ED nurses, internal medicine residents, internists, ED physicians, radiologists and laboratory assistants). It is important to achieve knowledge about everyone's professional interests. Finally, it is important to determine different subgroups in the group as a whole, mainly identifying the 'early adapters'. If these persons are also being respected by their colleagues they may fulfill the role of opinion leader or role model. To motivate and accompany the other subgroups in the sepsis protocol usage, the 'adapters' have to be involved in the implementation process actively.

III. Strategy of implementation

An implementation plan (including allocation of tasks) and a timetable have to be developed. The aims of the interventions should be: draw attention to the new protocol, stimulate active use of the new protocol in practice, and provide regular feedback of the results. The interventions should be aimed at health care workers, the ED organization, and material conditions.

Examples of possible interventions:

- To facilitate access to the protocol, make the sepsis protocol available to all employees using the intranet;
- Educate nurses, ED residents and internal medicine residents about sepsis and give information about the (content of the) sepsis protocol;
- Screening lists and registration forms should be available at the ED;
- Give ED nurses regular feedback on implementation issues;
- Emphasize the most relevant items of the sepsis protocol to the ED nurses;
- Utilize a nurse practitioner and/or medical student for data registration.

At first, the protocol has to be introduced to the target group. The first months after introduction of the protocol, the involved persons have to get familiar with the protocol and the registration of patients with sepsis. Subsequently, the nurses should get feedback on their performance of the recommendations. To provide the involved persons with insight in their own performance, changes in performance per recommendation can be presented during a department meeting. The effect of giving feedback should be evaluated after 3-4 months. If, after giving feedback, the performance of the protocol leaves much to be desired, inventory of promoting factors and barriers should be carried out.

IV. Evaluation

Short evaluations about the registration of data have to be planned periodically: for example once per 3-4 months. The evaluations provide an insight into the effects of the implementation strategies on the quality of care for patients with sepsis in the ED and it gives the opportunity to react to items that need more attention. Based on the evaluation, recommendations that were generally performed adequately and those that need more attention can be determined. Through interviewing the ED nurses, it is possible to carry out a more specified analysis of barriers in the performance of the sepsis protocol. Based on the interview results, adapted and/or new interventions can be described and applied. Herewith, the evaluation is a never ending process.

RESULTS OF IMPLEMENTATION STRATEGIES

Implementation of the Protocol

A total number of 825 patients $\geq$ 16 years visiting the ED, with (suspicion of) an infection and the presence of $\geq$ 2 extended SIRS criteria were included in our hospital. We measured the effects of our two-step implementation program: the introduction of a newly developed multidisciplinary sepsis registration protocol at the ED followed by education and feedback on compliance with the SSC recommendations for early recognition and treatment of septic patients. The performance of this implementation program resulted in an improved recognition and treatment of septic patients. Our multiple implementation activities resulted in significant changes in four out of six recommendations: (1) measure lactate $\leq$ 6 hours (from 23% to 80%), (2) perform a chest X-ray (from 67% to 83%), (3) take urine for urinalysis and culture (from 49% to 67%), and (4) start antibiotics $\leq$ 3 hours (from 38% to 56%). Taking two blood cultures before starting antibiotics did not improve significantly, probably caused by an already high score at baseline (from 83% to 86%). Also, the median time to hospitalization or discharge of the patient from the ED did not improve significantly. Compliance with the bundle of six recommendations improved significantly from 3.0 to 4.2 (improvement: 95%CI=0.9-1.5).

After the performance of different implementation activities, the following results were achieved:
- Clinical data of patients with sepsis in the ED are adequately registered;
- Compliance to the SSC guidelines improved strongly:

complete performance of diagnostics in more patients;

complete performance of diagnostics and therapeutic actions within the required time in more patients.

- Well performed separate issues:

triage of patients;

measure lactate;

take 2 blood cultures before start antibiotics;

take urine for urinalysis and culture;

perform a chest X-ray;

administration of antibiotics within 3 hours;

fill out the registration form completely.

Patient Characteristics That Influence the Compliance to the Protocol

The outcome of protocol adherence was expressed as the total number of recommendations that were correctly followed (0-6 scale). Through analyzing the compliance with the overall recommendation bundle for a group of 378 patients as a whole, it was proven that four different patient characteristics influenced the overall compliance rate significantly (both before and after protocol implementation): age, CRP result, intensive care unit admission, and the final diagnosis: every ten years increase of age demonstrated an increased overall score with 0.14 points. Furthermore, the mean overall compliance score for patients with a CRP result >150 was 0.4 points higher than the mean score for patients who had a CRP result <150 as well as the mean overall compliance score for patients admitted to the intensive care unit was 0.8 points higher than the mean score for patients who were not. Finally, in patients with a final diagnosis of pulmonary- or urinary tract infection, the overall performance scores, 4.4 and 4.6 respectively, were significantly higher ($P<0.001$) than the scores for patients with another focus of infection (3.9) or a non-infectious diagnosis.

Improving the Knowledge of Internal Medicine Residents

Following an educational intervention about sepsis, internal medicine residents' knowledge about sepsis definitions, and diagnosis and treatment of sepsis improved significantly [37]. One of the main findings of this study is that, apart from the short-term effects, the improved test results were sustained after 4-6 months. In the first (baseline) questionnaire, the issues relating to the sepsis definitions scored significantly lower than those related to the treatment of sepsis. This might be related to the fact that the Bone criteria [8], which are globally acknowledged and used, demonstrate a high sensitivity, but low specificity for sepsis and may not equal the clinical perception of the residents of a septic patient.

TOP 10 SUCCESSFUL IMPLEMENTATION TIPS

The following activities may contribute to successful implementation of a nurse-driven sepsis protocol in the ED:

1. Form a multidisciplinary team with motivated people;
2. Involve representatives from the target group in the implementation;
3. Spread the message;
4. Spread the message positively;
5. Do not break your engagements;
6. Be reachable;
7. Give your feedback in a positive way;
8. Also mention the well performed issues;
9. Be closely associated with the department, be visible on a regular basis;
10. Making a change is nearly always exciting!

CONCLUSION

The implementation of a protocol is difficult. The use of different, combined implementation strategies have to be used. The implementation of a predominantly nurse-driven sepsis registration protocol combined with education and feedback can significantly improve the recognition and treatment of patients with sepsis at the ED. Therefore, more attention should be given to the role of nurses in quality improvement of sepsis care. The influence of different patient characteristics on the overall compliance rate have to be explored and additional implementation strategies have to be focused on these influencing patient characteristics. To reach a sustained improved knowledge on symptoms, diagnosis and treatment of sepsis, different educational activities should be performed more often.

REFERENCES

[1]   Angus, DC; Linde-Zwirble, WT; Lidicker, J; Clermont, G; Carcillo, J; Pinsky, MR. Epidemiology of severe sepsis in the United States: analysis of incidence, outcome, and associated costs of care. Crit Care Med, 2001, 29(7), 1303-10.

[2]   Dellinger, RP; Levy, MM; Carlet, JM; Bion, J; Parker, MM; Jaeschke, R; et al. Surviving Sepsis Campaign: international guidelines for management of severe sepsis and septic shock: 2008. *Crit Care Med*, 2008, 36(1), 296-327.

[3]   Gao, F; Melody, T; Daniels, DF; Giles, S; Fox, S. The impact of compliance with 6-hour and 24-hour sepsis bundles on hospital mortality in patients with severe sepsis: a prospective observational study. *Crit Care*, 2005, 9(6), R764-R770.

[4]   Bone, RC. Sepsis, the sepsis syndrome, multi-organ failure: a plea for comparable definitions. *Ann Intern Med*, 1991, 114(4), 332-3.

[5]   Sibbald, WJ; Marshall, J; Christou, N; Girotti, M; McCormack, D; Rostein, O; et al. "Sepsis"--clarity of existing terminology ... or more confusion? *Crit Care Med*, 1991, 19(8), 996-8.

[6]   Bone, RC. Let's agree on terminology: definitions of sepsis. *Crit Care Med,* 1991, 19(7), 973-6.

[7]   Sprung, CL. Definitions of sepsis--have we reached a consensus? *Crit Care Med*, 1991, 19(7), 849-51.

[8]   Bone, RC; Balk, RA; Cerra, FB; Dellinger, RP; Fein, AM; Knaus, WA; et al. Definitions for sepsis and organ failure and guidelines for the use of innovative therapies in sepsis. The ACCP/SCCM Consensus Conference Committee. American College of Chest Physicians/Society of Critical Care Medicine. *Chest*, 1992, 101(6), 1644-55.

[9]   Nguyen, HB; Rivers, EP; Abrahamian, FM; Moran, GJ; Abraham, E; Trzeciak, S; et al. Severe sepsis and septic shock: review of the literature and emergency department management guidelines. *Ann Emerg Med*, 2006, 48(1), 28-54.

[10]   Rivers, EP; McIntyre, L; Morro, DC; Rivers, KK. Early and innovative interventions for severe sepsis and septic shock: taking advantage of a window of opportunity. *CMAJ*, 2005, 173(9), 1054-65.

[11]   Kumar, A; Roberts, D; Wood, KE; Light, B; Parrillo, JE; Sharma, S; et al. Duration of hypotension before initiation of effective antimicrobial therapy is the critical determinant of survival in human septic shock. *Crit Care Med*, 2006, 34(6), 1589-96.

[12]   Osborn, TM; Nguyen, HB; Rivers, EP. Emergency medicine and the surviving sepsis campaign: an international approach to managing severe sepsis and septic shock. *Ann Emerg Med*, 2005, 46(3), 228-31.

[13]   Dellinger, RP; Carlet, JM; Masur, H; Gerlach, H; Calandra, T; Cohen, J; et al. Surviving Sepsis Campaign guidelines for management of severe sepsis and septic shock. *Crit Care Med*, 2004, 32(3), 858-73.

[14]   Levy, MM; Fink, MP; Marshall, JC; Abraham, E; Angus, D; Cook, D; et al. 2001 SCCM/ESICM/ACCP/ATS/SIS International Sepsis Definitions Conference. *Crit Care Med*, 2003, 31(4), 1250-6.

[15]   Shapiro, N; Howell, MD; Bates, DW; Angus, DC; Ngo, L; Talmor, D. The association of sepsis syndrome and organ dysfunction with mortality in emergency department patients with suspected infection. *Ann Emerg Med*, 2006, 48(5), 583-90.

[16]   Annane, D; Bellissant, E; Cavaillon, JM. Septic shock. *Lancet*, 2005, 365(9453), 63-78.

[17]   Baldwin, LN; Smith, SA; Fender, V; Gisby, S; Fraser, J. An audit of compliance with the sepsis resuscitation care bundle in patients admitted to A&E with severe sepsis or septic shock. *Int Emerg Nurs*, 2008, 16(4), 250-6.

[18]   Micek, ST; Roubinian, N; Heuring, T; Bode, M; Williams, J; Harrison, C; et al. Before-after study of a standardized hospital order set for the management of septic shock. *Crit Care Med*, 2006, 34(11), 2707-13.

[19]   Shorr, AF; Micek, ST; Jackson, WL; Kollef, MH. Economic implications of an evidence-based sepsis protocol: can we improve outcomes and lower costs? *Crit Care Med*, 2007, 35(5), 1257-62.

[20]   Nguyen, HB; Corbett, SW; Steele, R; Banta, J; Clark, RT; Hayes, SR; et al. Implementation of a bundle of quality indicators for the early management of severe

sepsis and septic shock is associated with decreased mortality. *Crit Care Med*, 2007, 35(4), 1105-12.

[21] Carter, C. Implementing the severe sepsis care bundles outside the ICU by outreach. *Nurs Crit Care*, 2007, 12(5), 225-30.

[22] Robson, W; Beavis, S; Spittle, N. An audit of ward nurses' knowledge of sepsis. *Nurs Crit Care*, 2007, 12(2), 86-92.

[23] Grol, R. Successes and failures in the implementation of evidence-based guidelines for clinical practice. *Med Care*, 2001, 39(8 Suppl 2), II46-II54.

[24] Schuster, MA; McGlynn, EA; Brook, RH. How good is the quality of health care in the United States? 1998. *Milbank Q*, 2005, 83(4), 843-95.

[25] Grol, R; Grimshaw, J. From best evidence to best practice: effective implementation of change in patients' care. *Lancet*, 2003, 362(9391), 1225-30.

[26] Grol, R. Development of guidelines for general practice care. *Br J Gen Pract*, 1993, 43(369), 146-51.

[27] Burgers, JS; Grol, RP; Zaat, JO; Spies, TH; van der Bij, AK; Mokkink, HG. Characteristics of effective clinical guidelines for general practice. *Br J Gen Pract*, 2003, 53(486),15-9.

[28] Grol, RP; Bosch, MC; Hulscher, ME; Eccles, MP; Wensing, M. Planning and studying improvement in patient care: the use of theoretical perspectives. *Milbank Q*, 2007, 85(1), 93-138.

[29] Grimshaw, JM; Thomas, RE; Maclennan, G; Fraser, C; Ramsay, CR; Vale, L; et al. Effectiveness and efficiency of guideline dissemination and implementation strategies. *Health Technol Assess*, 2004, 8(6), iii-iv,1-72.

[30] Wensing, M; Wollersheim, H; Grol, R. Organizational interventions to implement improvements in patient care: a structured review of reviews. *Implement Sci*, 2006, 1:2.

[31] Grol, R; Wensing, M; Eccles, MP. *Improving patient care. The Implementation of Change in Clinical Practice*. Edinburgh: Elsevier Butterworth Heinemann; 2004.

[32] Cabana, MD; Rand, CS; Powe, NR; Wu, AW; Wilson, MH; Abboud, PA; et al. Why don't physicians follow clinical practice guidelines? A framework for improvement. *JAMA*, 1999, 282(15), 1458-65.

[33] Carlbom, DJ; Rubenfeld, GD. Barriers to implementing protocol-based sepsis resuscitation in the emergency department--results of a national survey. *Crit Care Med*, 2007, 35(11), 2525-32.

[34] Baiardini, I; Braido, F; Bonini, M; Compalati, E; Canonica, GW. Why do doctors and patients not follow guidelines? *Curr Opin Allergy Clin Immunol*, 2009, 9(3), 228-33.

[35] Fernandez, R; Galera, A; Rodriguez, W; Rive-Mora, E; Rodriguez-Vega, G. Sepsis: a study of physician's knowledge about the surviving sepsis campaign in Puerto Rico. *Crit Care & Shock*, 2007, 10(4), 131-41.

[36] Ziglam, HM; Morales, D; Webb, K; Nathwani, D. Knowledge about sepsis among training-grade doctors. *J Antimicrob Chemother*, 2006, 57(5), 963-5.

[37] Tromp, M; Bleeker-Rovers, CP; Achterberg van, T; Kullberg, BJ; Hulscher, M; Pickkers, P. Internal medicine residents' knowledge about sepsis: Effects of a teaching intervention. Neth J Med, 2009, 67(9), 312-5.

In: Sepsis: Symptoms, Diagnosis and Treatment
Editor: Joseph R. Brown, pp. 107-127
ISBN: 978-1-60876-609-3
© 2010 Nova Science Publishers, Inc.

Chapter 6

APOPTOSIS IN SEPSIS

Stefan Weber[1], Stephanie Brümmer-Smith[2] and Stefan Schröder[3]*

[1]Dept. of Anesthesiology and Intensive Care Medicine, University of Bonn Medical
Center, Sigmund-Freud-Str. 25, D-53105 Bonn, Germany
[2]Dep. of Intensive Care Medicine, Guy's and St Thomas' Hospital,
Lambeth Palace Road, London SE 1 7EH
[3]Dept. of Anesthesiology and Intensive Care Medicine, West Coast Hosptial,
Esmarchstr. 50, D-25746 Heide, Germany

ABSTRACT

Sepsis is a leading cause of death in many intensive care units. The pathophysiology is characterized by a dysregulation of the immune system in response to infection or secondary to a trauma. Initial hyperinflammation often results in septic shock.. Simultaneously, part of the immune system is deactivated leading to a temporary but often deadly immunosuppression. Recently, apoptosis of immunocompetent cells is being recognized as a key mechanism in the immunosuppression during sepsis. There is mounting evidence both in murine models and human patients, that apoptosis of lymphocytes, monocytes and dentritic cells is accelerated already in the early phases of sepsis. Inhibition of apoptosis in mouse models of sepsis by pan-caspase inhibition improves survival. Current studies suggest a role of both death receptors and the mitochondria in the initiation of apoptosis. Blocking the death receptor pathway with a fusion protein against Fas or by silencing the downstream caspase 8 results in a reduction of mortality after experimental induction of sepsis. On the other hand, protection of the mitochondrial integrity by over expression of the antiapoptotic protein bcl-2 improves survival as well. In humans, both an upregulation of Fas and a downregulation of bcl-2 are observed in lymphocytes of patients suffering from severe sepsis. In conclusion, the inhibition of accelerated apoptosis during sepsis is a promising target in the design of a novel and specific immunotherapy of sepsis.

---

* Corresponding author: E-mail: stefan.weber@ukb.uni-bonn.de

INTRODUCTION

There is mounting evidence that sepsis and the systemic inflammatory response syndrome (SIRS) are immunological disorders, and that apoptosis of leukocytes contributes significantly to the pathophysiology of sepsis. Sepsis and SIRS are characterized by the inability of the immune system to contain the inflammation within one site (Figure 1). Instead, the body responds with a systemic inflammation to a local stimulus, such as bacterial, fungal or viral infection, but also surgical trauma. The initial hyperinflammation very soon is accompanied by an anti-inflammatory modulation of the immunsystem in an attempt to counterbalance the excessive inflammatory load. Massive activation- and deactivation signalling ultimately results in a dysbalanced immune system. In this phase, critically ill patients often succumb to secondary infections. The complete mechanisms of the temporary immunosupression during systemic inflammatory disorders is yet unresolved, however convincing evidence attributes apoptosis of leukocytes a prominent role.

The first part of this chapter focuses on the definition, epidemiology and pathophysiology of the diseases sepsis and SIRS. In the second part, mechanisms of apoptosis are explained. The third part finally reviews current research on the role of apoptosis in sepsis and SIRS.

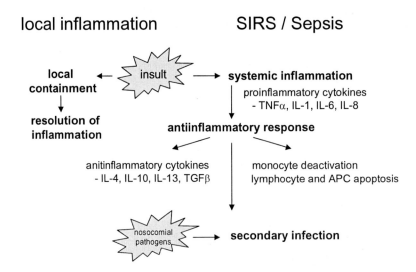

Figure 1. Immunological response pattern of sepsis / SIRS: Failure to contain the response to a local insult (bacteria, fungi, virus or trauma) results in systemic inflammation and as a consequence to the production of anti-inflammatory cytokines, the deactivation of antigen presenting cells (APC's) and apoptosis of APC's and lymphocytes.

Table 1. Diagnostic Criteria for SIRS

- body temperature >38°C or <35°C
- heart rate >90 beats per minute
- tachypnoea >20 per minute or hyperventilation with p_aCO_2<32 mmHg
- leukozytosis >12,0 x 10^9 cells/l or leukopenia < 4,0 x 10^9 cells/l or >10% stab neutrophils

2 or more criteria need to be fulfilled to diagnose SIRS.

DEFINITION OF SEPSIS AND IMMUNOLOGICAL PROCESSES

Epidemiology

Despite recent advances in medicine sepsis remains one of the leading causes of death in critically ill patients. The Systemic Inflammatory Response Syndrome (SIRS)occurs in up to 80% of that patient group and up to30% will progress to sepsis. A further 10-15% will develop severe sepsis and multiple organ failure (MOF) [1]. According to a paper by Brun-Buisson the overall mortality for sepsis ranges around 20 % and up 40-60% for patients with septic shock[1]. According to estimations within the United States there is a prevalence of 3 cases per 1000 citizens acquiring sepsis each year and 2.6 cases of sepsis for each patient leaving hospital. In America the average morbidity is 28,6% and increases up to 38.5% for patients above 85 years of age. The overall costs for treating sepsis run at 16.7 million dollars US per annum , 22.000 $ per case. Since 1995 the incidence has been steadily increasing by 1.5 % per year[2;3]. In Germany, a recent survey of the SepNet study group reported a 54% mortality in severe sepsis[4;5]. A French multicentred study revealed that most cases of sepsis are nosocomial, up to 25% are acquired within the critical care setting [6].

Definitions

For SIRS to be diagnosed two or more specific criteria need to be met (Table 1). Whereas SIRS can be caused by non-infectious events like trauma, burns, pancreatitis etc, sepsis is defined as being caused by any form of infective organisms or a strong suspicion for infection [7; 8].These definitions for SIRS and sepsis are about to be challenged by the new PIRO concept, developed at the Consensus Conference held in Toronto, Ont., Canada in 2001. PIRO is an anagram where P is predisposition, I is infection, R stands for response and O for organ dysfunction [9-13].

Pathophysiology of the Immune Response

The mainstay of sepsis therapy remains symptomatic treatment with haemodynamic and organ support, as well as aggressive treatment of underlying infection with antibiotics or surgical intervention[14;15]. During sepsis the host response is an array of complex immunological processes, which are partially self-perpetuating and partially inhibitory with regards to the immune response[16]. It thus makes sense to look for possible therapeutic interventions that modulate the innate immune response[17]. But a detailed and thorough knowledge of processes involved is necessary. During sepsis immuncompetent cells are activated. The activation of leukocytes and the inflammatory response take place in a generalised pattern, not limited to specific body compartments. The first phase during sepsis is called "hyperinflammatory phase" and is characterised by an excessive production of proinflammatory cytokines, e.g tumor necrosis factor-α (TNF-α), interleukin 1 (IL-1), interleukin-6 (IL-6) and interleukin-8 (IL-8)[18]. Parallel to an inflammatory reaction there is also production of anti-inflammatory cytokines[17]. Namely interleukin-10 (IL-10), transforming-growth-factor-β, interleukin-13 (IL-13), interleukin-4 (IL-4) and platelet-activating-factor (PAF). An excessive production of anti-inflammatory cytokines can lead to a process termed "immunoparalysis", whereby the host response to infection and infective organisms is inadequate[19]. This can lead to an exacerbation of the septic process. A detailed description of the cytokine cascade can be found elsewhere[20;21]. In conjunction with a more detailed understanding of immunphysiological processes during sepsis over the last years, apoptosis has been recognized as one of the key factors in the pathophysiology of sepsis. Accelerated apoptosis seems to be induced in leukocytes and many immuncompetent cells during sepsis, as shown in several animal models[22;23]. In humans similar processes are involved[24].

At this point, it is important to note, that neutrophil apoptosis is regulateted very differently during sepsis. In contrast to most other leukocytes, neutrophil apoptosis is markedly downregulated.[25-27].

Inhibition of apoptosis in a mouse model did dramatically improve survival[28], which proves that the process of apoptosis is involved in the regulation of the immune response during sepsis. This might open up the way for new novel immunmodulating therapies[29]. We will now describe the basic underlying mechanisms of apoptosis and then explain several investigations looking at apoptosis during sepsis in animal models. Finally we will present an overview on the current status of human studies into apoptosis in septic patients and their possible implications for future therapies.

MOLECULAR MECHANISM OF APOPTOSIS

Overall organised cell death is as important as proliferation and mitosis in human beings to maintain a balance between organised cell growth and death. The human body contains about 10^{14} cells, each of which is able to initiate apoptosis [30]. Every day there are about 60 x 10^9 newly developing cells. Old ones get removed by programmed cell death and other processes[31]. In 1972 Kerr, Curie et al introduced the term apoptosis to characterizes a form of programmed cell death that exhibited a specific morphology[32;33]. They distinguished apoptosis from necrosis and presumed that the process of apoptosis was based on a genetically encoded programme. Apoptosis seemed to happen in an orderly fashion in healthy tissue, normal development and tumor regression. Over the last 30 years it has been shown that apoptosis goes back to early primitive life forms and seems to be found in nematode *Caenorhabditis elegans* as well as in human beings[34]. Even during embryonic development apoptosis in certain cells is vital to eliminate or reorganise structures, eg the elimination of interdigital folds and thymus atrophy[35]. The principal function of programmed cell death is to create a balance between cell mitosis, growth and cell death. Thus major organs and the immunsystem get regenerated while the overall cell number remains fairly constant[31]. In the adult human being apoptosis plays an important role for the elimination of damaged non-functional cells. Apoptosis also is a key factor during oncogenesis. Programmed cell death should normally occur in mutated cells and eliminate potential tumor cells. Malignant cells do however find many ways to circumvent those mechanisms and escape cell death[36]. It is know that in malignant melanoma several mutations allow tumor cells to escape the death-receptor mediated elimination via apoptosis[37].

Morphology

Apoptosis is characterised by sequential changes which are different from processes during necrosis (Table 2). Initially there is cell-volume reduction. Intracellular organelles as well as intracellular metabolism remain intact[38]. There is shrinkage of the nucleus and condensation of chromatin (pyknosis). Specific calcium and magnesium dependent DNAses become activated and cleave the DNA into fragments [39]. The plasma membrane produces pseudopodia containing nuclear fragments and organelles. These break off into several membrane-bound vesicles in a process called "membrane blebbing"[38].While the cytoplasmatic membrane remains intact, those apoptotic bodies break off. Characteristic for programmed cell death is that single apoptotic cells can be found amongst otherwise normal cells, whereas necrosis involves multiple surrounding cells. During necrosis the cell and organelles swell which ultimately causes membrane rupture. Lysosomal enzymes break down intracellular structures. An array of highly reactive species like cytokines, free radicals and enzymes get released which cause an influx of neutrophils and macrophages, leading to a generalised inflammation[40]. In apoptosis however potential proinflammatory molecules become compartmentalised so that there is no concurrent inflammatory response. Apoptotic cells are able to express molecules like phosphatidylcholin on their cell surface, marking the cell for phagocytosis by macrophages[41]. This mechanism builds the basis for a selective organised elimination of cells, preventing a local inflammation of the surrounding tissue[38]. Apart from the traditional process of apoptosis there is a third process, which is different to necrosis, but also does not meet all criteria for apoptosis[42-45]. It is either called apoptosis-like or necrosis-like programmed cell death. This process depicts different intracellular signalling cascades[38], for example the apoptosis inducing factor AIF[46]{Mate, Ortiz-Lombardia, et al. 2002.

Caspase Cascade

The main effectors of apoptosis are a family of protein degrading enzymes, called caspases (CASP)[34]. They are proenzymes that have been conserved from nematodes to humans. Fourteen human caspases have been described so far. They all have the aminoacid cystein in their active centrum and cleave substrates off after aspartate[47] Depending on the steric conformation in the active centre the substrate specifity is determined. During the initiator phase death signals are taken up by caspases, a process that initiates apoptosis[34;48]. A cascade of events leads to further activation of effectorcaspases and finally the degradation of relevant proteins (effector and degradation phase).

Initiatorphase

Taking the CD95-initiated apoptosis as an example figure one depicts a typical signalling pathway. CD59 (Fas) and tumornecrosisfactor-α-receptor are so called death receptors. They are transmembrane glycoproteins which are situated in the cell membrane[49]. The Fas-receptor is activated by binding of Fas-ligand (Fas-L) that is located on the surface of lymphocyte subsets. It subsequently leads to intracellular production of adaptation molecules, which are termed Fas-associated death domain (FADD) and procaspase-8, which is recruited to the receptor[50]. procaspase 8 gets cleaved to caspase-8 and thus activated . It is then able to activate caspase-3 by splicing off a fragment of procaspase-3[34]. Caspase-3 is responsible for degrading structural and functional proteins and initiating apaotosis[34]. Overall the Fas pathway is important in controlling apoptosis and the immune response, e.g. the activation induced cell death of lymphocytes[51].

Effectorphase

Caspase-3 is responsible for activating the enzyme Caspase-Activated-DNAse (CAD), which splits the DNA into characteristic fragments[52;53]. Zeiosis, a change in the plasmamembrane is caused by digestion of the cytoskeleton through caspase-3[54;55]. Caspases also activate an enzyme called scramblase, which externalises phosphatidylserin onto the membrane surface and thus marks cells for phagocytosis[40;56].

Mitochondrial Pathway

A second apoptotic pathway, mitochondrial-dependent apoptosis, occurs in response to a variety of injurious stimuli. The mitochondrium contains multiple pro-apoptotic molecules which can amplify the incoming apoptotic signal[57]. A caspase-8 mediated cleavage of protein Bid to truncated protein Bid (tBid) transfers the signal to the mitochondria[58]. Regulatory molecules belonging to the Bcl-2 family are situated in the outer mitochondrial membrane. They regulate the activation of pro-apoptotic molecules. They may for example protect the cells from death induced by cytotoxic agents. There are at least 25 members of the bcl-2 family[59]. Whereas group I molecules like Bcl-2 are anti-apoptotic, group II molecules like Bax and group III molecules like Bis are pro-apoptotic[58]. All proteins interact with each other and influence regulation and release of further signalling molecules. One possible mechanism is the opening and closure of the mitochondrial "permeability transition pore complex"[60]. It leads to the release of cytochrome c, caspase-9 and the adaptor protein Apaf-1 into the cytosol. Together they from a multienzymecomplex, the so called apoptosom. It interlinks with the caspase cascade by activating caspase-3[34]. In order to prevent unintended cell death a number of complex feedbackmechanisms exist regulate the signalling pathways of apoptosis[61]. An example are the "inhibitor of apoptosis proteins" (IAP's)[62],which themselves are regulated by the mitochondrial protein Smac-Diablo[63].

APOPTOSIS IN SEPSIS

Apoptosis can be induced by multiple mechanisms and cells vary in their specific response. Nonetheless apoptosis seems to be the final common pathway in septic processes after activation of different signalling transduction pathways. Apoptosis has been shown to be a major factor in several animal models of sepsis[28;64-79]. In humans only few studies looked at the role of apoptosis during sepsis[80-84]. Studies of apoptosis in human sepsis are hampered by the complex interactions during sepsis and a complex time course of pro- and anti-inflammatory events. The other problem is the multifactorial ethiology which makes it difficult to attribute certain events to a specific process.

A recent study by Henriksson puts forward an interesting link between apoptosis and the coagulations system. It is well known that the complex dysregulation is one of the main culprits of organ dysfunction in sepsis[85]. He and his group observed that non-viable endotoxin-treated monocytes are strongly procoagulant[86]. This effect was not only dependent on the expression of tissue factor, a well-known inducer but also on the presence of externalised phosphatidyl serin. Since phosphatidyl serin is externalised on apoptotic cells, excessive apoptosis of circulating cells may act as a procoagulant and thus further worsen the course of sepsis and promote organ failure.

Another startling finding the fact that adoptive transfer of apoptotic splenocytes worsens survival, whereas adoptive transfer of necrotic splenocytes improves survival in sepsis[87]. A possible explanation of this observation is the effect of apoptotic cells on macrophages. Ingestion of apoptotic cells not only fails to induce an inflammatory response but actually elicits an antiinflammatory response. This response may cause further immunosupression and thus set the stage for secondary infections.

Increased Apoptosis in Leukocyte Subsets

Accelerated apoptosis during sepsis has been detected in diverse immunocompetent cell types.

Among them, lymphocytes play a critical role[28].B-lymphocyte[68;83] as well as CD4+[69] and CD8+ T-cells[84] undergo apoptosis in response to sepsis. Suprisingly, even though the percentage of CD4+CD25+ regulatory T-lymphocytes increases during sepsis, regulatory T-cells undergo accelerated apoptosis[88]. The increased ratio can be explained by the even more increased apoptosis rate of CD4+CD25+ T-cells. Natural killer (NK) cells are known to play in important role in the control of cancer cells. In a model of systemic inflammation by administration of IL-2 and IL-12, NK-cells underwent rapid apoptosis[89]. No alteration in regard to apoptosis during sepsis has been observed so far in the subset of deltagamma T-lymphocytes. Still, a lack of deltagamma T-lymphocytes worsens the outcome of sepsis and contributes to immunosupression[90]. Moreover, accelerated apoptosis has been detected in monocytes[91], dendritic cells [82;92;93], thymocytes[23;75;94] and bone marrow[22]. Apart from the progressive loss of dendritic cells, surviving dendritic cells mature rapidly but fail to initiate a protective Th-1 type immune response.

Apoptosis in Animal Models

Initially experiments in animals where used to examine general principles and signalling cascades of apoptosis. Recent investigations have been extended to animal models of sepsis. It is common practice to use ligation and perforation of the coecum to cause bacterial peritonitis (CLP model)[78;95]. Apoptosis has been linked to the severity of sepsis. In the

CLP model signs of apoptosis could be found in thymus, lung and intestinal mucosa and epithelium[78]. Investigations in a mouse model showed that there seems to be a TNF and endotoxin- independent stimulation of apoptosis[96;96]. Animal models also show, that lymphocyte apoptosis in sepsis is mostly independent of p53 [74].

Caspase-Cascade

Several animal models have been used to examine the role of specific apoptotic signalling cascades. Caspases-3,-6 and-9 but not caspase-1 are activated in sepsis induced thymocyte apoptosis[75]. Overexpression of caspases seems to induce apoptosis[97], whereas certain caspase inhibitors like the viral cowpox-encoded protein CmA are able to prevent apoptosis[98]. Inhibition of apoptosis confers a survival benefit in CLP-induced sepsis[18]. Three different mechanisms have been tested: Application of a broad-spectrum caspase inhibitor z-VAD, that blocks some but not all caspases, M 920, an inhibitor of caspases-1,-3 and -8, as well as M-971 a selective inhibitor of caspase-3 which leads to inhibition of lymphocytic apoptosis[28;76]. Consequently, treated mice had a higher survival rate secondary to enhanced immunity. Preventing caspase-3 activation with genetic engineering shows similar effects and Caspase-3-deficient mice have a significant higher survival rate in CLP-induced sepsis[28]. The inhibition of caspase-11 by knock out improves survival of sepsis in a murine model[99]. Also, the lack of caspase-12 conferred resistance to experimentally induced sepsis in mice and improved the bacterial clearance[100].

Fas Induced Apoptosis

Several lines of evidence support an important role of the death receptor Fas in accelerated leukocyte apoptosis during sepsis[101]. Increased inducible apoptosis in CD4+ T lymphocytes during polymicrobial sepsis is mediated by Fas ligand[69], because FasL-deficient C3H/HeJ-Fasl gld mice are more resistant to apoptosis after CLP. Blocking of the Fas-FasL-system by the application of a Fas-receptor fusion protein also decreased apoptosis during polymicrobial sepsis[102].

Fas activated its downstream caspase-8 by recruiting it to the death domain. The knock-down of functional caspase-8 by an *in vivo* siRNA approach improved the survival of septic mice[70].

Mitochondrial Pathway

As explained earlier, apoptosis may not only be induced by death receptors, but also by the release of proapoptotic factors from the mitochondrium[60;103]. As far as the mitochondrial apoptotic pathway is concerned, T-cells with overexpression of bcl-2 are completely protected against sepsis-induced T-lymphocyte apoptosis in lymphatic tissue like thymus and spleen[77] . Other investigations support these findings, demonstrating a reduced lymphocytic apoptosis with bcl-2 overexpression. The survival benefit reached up to fifty percent[76]. When a BclXL-fusion protein or a BH4-domain-fusion protein were introduced in the CLP-model apoptosis was reduced and survival improved [104]. The survival kinase AKT can influence the transcription of proteins of the bcl-2 family. Overexpression of AKT in a murine CLP-model improved survival and boostered the Th-1 cytokine response with an increase in interferon-γ and decrease in IL-4[79]. However, this effect was independent of blc-2[79].

Neutrophil Apoptosis

Although neutropenia after chemotherapy or as the result of a genetic defect[105-109] threatens the life of patients, an excessive amount of active neutrophils contributes to the organ damage observed in sepsis[110]. Neutrophils produce a variety of toxic compounds that not only exterminate pathogens but also damage surrounding tissue[111]. The normal life span of a neutrophil is rather short. They last for less than a day within the circulation. In contrast to most other leukocytes, neutrophil apoptosis is delayed in sepsis[112]. The inhibition of neutrophil apoptosis is induced by proinflammatory cytokines and may be counteracted by IL-10[113]. Within the cell the mitochondrial pathway seems to be involved. Delayed neutrophil apoptosis in sepsis is associated with maintenance of mitochondrial transmembrane potential, retention of cytochrome c in the mitochondrion and as a consequence a reduced caspase-9 activity[27].

Apoptosis in Other Cells and Organs

Even though the main focus of this review are leukocytes, it is nevertheless important to point out, that also other cell types undergo accelerated apoptosis in sepsis. These phenomena may contribute profoundly to the development of multiple organ failure during sepsis.

Intestines: Several investigators have shown a major role of the intestinal epithelium in the pathophysiology of sepsis[114-116]. Often the gut is considered the "motor" of SIRS and sepsis. Apoptosis in intestinal epithelial cells could be shown in several animal models[78;117]. A CLP-mouse-model with transgenic mice, which were overexpressing bcl-2 demonstrated a survival benefit of 39 % (83% after 8 days versus 44% in normal mice) (64). The same group investigated animals with sepsis due to Pseudomonas aeruginosa pneumonia. They showed a clear survival benefit in animals with overexpression of bcl-2 and subsequently reduced apoptosis of intestinal epithelial cells[118].

Heart: Many patients develop a cardiac dysfunction during sepsis. Current evidence implicates a role of cardiomyocyte apoptosis in the pathology of the septic shock heart[119]. Although cardiac myocytes are relatively resistant to apoptosis[120], a study by Lancel et al. suggests that an endotoxin-induced apoptotic pathway contributes significantly to sublethal, cytophatic changes in the heart [121;122]. Still the question remains to which extent actual apoptosis contributes to cardiac dysfunction[123], as is may not be the cell death itself, that is responsible. Carlson and his colleagues demonstrated, that endotoxin activates the apoptotic pathway via the TNF-receptor[124]. Inhibition of the caspases improved ventricular function. Since only low levels of apoptosis were observed at the time of ventricular dysfunction, another effect of caspases rather than the induction of apoptosis may be the reason for the observed defects[123]. Isolated left ventricular cardiomyocytes display decreased contractility in response to LPS-treatment. In a study by Lancel and his group, this was accompanied by an increased activity of caspases -3, -6 and -9. Pan-caspase inhibition prevented the contractile dysfunction, troponin T cleavage and sarcomere destruction[121].

Lung: In acute lung injury hallmarks beside acute neutrophilic alveolitis include the destruction of alveolar capillary epithelium [125]. Lung epithelial cells are subject to induced apoptosis[112]. The Fas/Fas-Ligand system seem to play a causal role in these events[126;127].

Liver: In the liver the inhibition of Fas increases hepatic blood flow and improves survival in sepsis[67].

Endothelium: Whether apoptosis of epithelial cells during the septic process is beneficial or rather harmful remains unclear at present[128].

APOPTOSIS IN HUMAN STUDIES

In serum of human patients with sepsis and SIRS, elevated levels of nucleosomes, a sign of late apoptosis are found[129]. The mRNA-expression of the antiapoptotic protein bcl-2 was transiently downregulated in patients with severe sepsis[130]. These are strong arguments for the involvement of apoptosis in human sepsis.

A prospective study looking at 20 septic patients who died of multiple organ failure demonstrated ongoing apoptosis in all patients. Histopathophysiologically apoptosis was predominantly found in intestinal epithelium (colon, ileum) and spleen [77]. Almost all septic patients had significant peripheral lymphocytopenia and also a reduction in lymphocytes in the spleen. The findings were interpreted as an indirect sign of lymphocytic apoptosis. As there was an increased splenic caspase-3 –activity, it was conferred to be a caspase–3-mediated apoptosis. This leads to a decreased immundefense in sepsis. Further investigations found focal apoptosis in gut tissue of ten trauma patients. Apoptotic foci were seen shortly after the traumatic insult in intestinal lymphoid and epithelial tissue[83]. A prospective study looking at 27 septic patients and 25 trauma patients demonstrated a Caspase-9 mediated reduction of B-and CD4-T-helper cells. Interestingly there was no reduction of CD8-positive T-cells or natural killer cells[83]. In spleens of patients with sepsis and trauma, a profound loss of dendritic cells but not macrophages was observed[82]. Since dendritic cells constitute the main pool of antigen presenting cells, an impaired activation of T- and B-cells may be expected[82].

Lymphocytes not only undergo accelerated apoptosis during sepsis but are also more responsive to secondary induction of apoptosis: Lymphocytes are more sensitive to activation induced cell death[80]. An increased apoptosis and subsequent loss of CD4-positive cells and B-cells seems paradoxical, as it occurs during a life threatening illness where rather an increase of all lymphocytes would be expected. Moreover, lymphocytes from septic patients proliferate less in response to Lectins or CD3[131].

Monocytes have been shown to respond with an increased expression of heat-shock-protein 70 (HSP 70) in septic patients[91]. This study looking at 18 septic patients and 17 healthy volunteers, also measured a reduced mitochondrial membrane potential which is an indicator of initiated irreversible monocyte apoptosis. Overall no difference could be found with regards to Bcl-2 concentration in septic and healthy patients. Sepsis survivors however had a significantly higher Bcl-2 concentration than non-survivors during the first 3 days [91].

Soluble modulators of apoptosis are markedly altered during sepsis. In paediatric sepsis soluble Fas (sFas) was increased, whereas soluble Fas Ligand (sFasL) was not[132]. In adult patients with sepsis sFas was elevated and was associated with poor survival[133]. In SIRS and sepsis sFas was found to be elevated by the group of Torre. However, in this study sFas did not correlate with the outcome[134]. sFas is believed to act as a scavenger of sFasL or as a dummy receptor of FasL on apoptosis-inducing cells. In this regard, an increase in sFas during sepsis may be interpreted as a compensatory mechanism to limit increased apoptosis.

In a study by De Freitas et al., serum levels of sFasL were elevated[135]. sFasL may act as an inducer of apoptosis in Fas bearing cells. This finding hints at the role of the Fas-FasL system in sepsis. The increase of soluble components may be due to endotoxaemia, because after endotoxaemia of healthy volunteers, an increase of sFAS as well as sFasL was detected [136]. The expression of Fas on monocytes after endotoxaemia was transiently downregulated but increased several fold within 24h[137]. In sepsis Fas and FasL were upregulated on lymphocytes in septic patients[81].

CONCLUSION

Although most studies looked at small patient numbers, it can be said that apoptosis plays an integral part in the pathophysiology of sepsis. A reduction in T-cell numbers caused by apoptosis may lead to immunsupression, which is potentially fatal[28]. A loss and dysfunction of APC's due to apoptosis probably results in a lack of T-cell activation[92;138]. Furthermore, the presence of apoptotic cells in the circulation may elicit a Th2-response, which acts rather antiinflammatory[87]. Lastly, posphatidyl and tissue factor bearing circulating apoptotic cells may act as a procoagulant and may further worsen the coagulation imbalance, hereby promoting organ failure[86].

On the other hand lymphocytic apoptosis may confer a survival benefit under specific circumstances by downregulating an overshooting inflammatory cascade. Neutrophils may cause harm in the acute inflammatory situation, but they are a key player in the resolution of inflammation, e.g. in the lung.

It will be important to discover more about the exact sequence of enzyme cascades and mediator release during the time course of sepsis to be able to target specific interactions. How apoptosis in parenchymal cells contributes to the development of multiple organ failure remains unclear and warrants further investigation. We do not know whether apoptosis is the cause of multi-organ-dysfunctions syndrome or whether it is an epiphenomenon. Looking at present investigations it is neither exactly known to which extent sepsis induces apoptosis in humans, nor during which specific phase apoptosis of lymphocytes occurs.

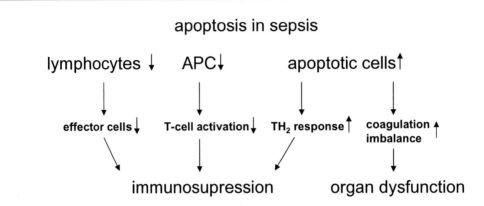

Figure 2. Potentially detrimental effects of apoptosis during sepsis

Specifically apoptosis in immuncompetent cells seems to offer the possibility to use potential diagnostic and therapeutic interventions in the future[29;139-141]. Possible approaches include the use of caspase inhibitors[28], antiapoptotic bcl-2 family fusion proteins[104] or the use of siRNA approach against caspases[70]. New concepts in the treatment of sepsis will only be successful if they take the exact timecourse of pro-and anti-inflammatory events into account, as well as looking at the timely events during apoptosis and their pathophysiological relevance.

REFERENCES

[1]   Brun-Buisson C. The epidemiology of the systemic inflammatory response. Intensive Care Med. 2000, 26 Suppl 1, S64-S74.

[2]   Angus, DC; Wax, RS. Epidemiology of sepsis: an update. *Crit. Care Med.*, 2001, 29(7 Suppl), S109-S116.

[3]   Angus, DC; Linde-Zwirble, WT; Lidicker, J; Clermont, G; Carcillo, J; Pinsky, MR. Epidemiology of severe sepsis in the United States: analysis of incidence, outcome, and associated costs of care. *Crit. Care Med.*, 2001, 29(7), 1303-1310.

[4]   Bauer, M; Brunkhorst, F; Welte, T; Gerlach, H; Reinhart, K. [Sepsis : Update on pathophysiology, diagnostics and therapy.] Sepsis: Aktuelle Aspekte zu Pathophysiologie, Diagnostik und Therapie. *Anaesthesist*, 2006 Jun 30, 2006.

[5]   Brunkhorst, FM. [Epidemiology, economy and practice -- results of the German study on prevalence by the competence network sepsis (SepNet)] Epidemiologie, Okonomie und Praxis -- Ergebnisse der deutschen Pravalenzstudie des Kompetenznetzwerkes Sepsis (SepNet). *Anasthesiol Intensivmed Notfallmed Schmerzther*, 2006 Jan; 41(1), 43 -4 2006, 41:43-44.

[6]   Brun-Buisson, C; Doyon, F; Carlet, J; Dellamonica, P; Gouin, F; Lepoutre, A; Mercier, JC; Offenstadt, G; Regnier, B. Incidence, risk factors, and outcome of severe sepsis and septic shock in adults. A multicenter prospective study in intensive care units. French ICU Group for Severe Sepsis. *JAMA*, 1995, 274(12), 968-974.

[7]   Bone, RC; Balk, RA; Cerra, FB; Dellinger, RP; Fein, AM; Knaus, WA; Schein, RM; Sibbald, WJ. Definitions for sepsis and organ failure and guidelines for the use of

innovative therapies in sepsis. The ACCP/SCCM Consensus Conference Committee. American College of Chest Physicians/Society of Critical Care Medicine. *Chest*, 1992, 101(6), 1644-1655.

[8]   Bone, RC. Sir Isaac Newton, sepsis, SIRS, and CARS. *Crit. Care Med.*, 1996, 24(7), 1125-1128.

[9]   Vincent, JL; Wendon, J; Groeneveld, J; Marshall, JC; Streat, S; Carlet, J. The PIRO concept: O is for organ dysfunction. *Crit. Care*, 2003 Jun, 7 (3), 260 -4 Epub 2003 May 7 2003, 7, 260-264.

[10]   Gerlach, H; Dhainaut, JF; Harbarth, S; Reinhart, K; Marshall, JC; Levy, M. The PIRO concept: R is for response. *Crit Care*, 2003 Jun, 7 (3), 256 -9 Epub 2003 May 8 2003, 7, 256-259.

[11]   Vincent, JL; Opal, S; Torres, A; Bonten, M; Cohen, J; Wunderink, R. The PIRO concept: I is for infection. *Crit.* Care 2003 Jun, 7(3), 252 -5 Epub 2003 May 7 2003, 7, 252-255.

[12]   Angus, DC; Burgner, D; Wunderink, R; Mira, JP; Gerlach, H; Wiedermann, CJ; Vincent, JL. The PIRO concept: P is for predisposition. *Crit Care*, 2003 Jun, 7(3), 248 - 51 Epub 2003 May 8 2003, 7, 248-251.

[13]   Levy, MM; Fink, MP; Marshall, JC; Abraham, E; Angus, D; Cook, D; Cohen, J; Opal, SM; Vincent, JL; Ramsay, G. 2001 SCCM/ESICM/ACCP/ATS/SIS International Sepsis Definitions Conference. *Crit Care Med*, 2003, 31(4), 1250-1256.

[14]   Meier-Hellmann, A; Bredle, DL; Reinhart, K. Treating patients with severe sepsis. *N. Engl. J. Med.*, 1999, 341, 56.

[15]   Wheeler, AP; Bernard, GR. Treating patients with severe sepsis. *N. Engl. J. Med.*, 1999, 340, 207-214.

[16]   Cohen, J. The immunopathogenesis of sepsis. *Nature*, 2002 Dec 2002, 420, 885-891.

[17]   Kox, WJ; Volk, T; Kox, SN; Volk, HD. Immunomodulatory therapies in sepsis. *Intensive Care Med.*, 2000, 26 Suppl 1, S124-S128.

[18]   Hotchkiss, RS; Karl, IE. The pathophysiology and treatment of sepsis. *N Engl J Med*, 2003, 348(2), 138-150.

[19]   Docke, WD; Randow, F; Syrbe, U; Krausch, D; Asadullah, K; Reinke, P; Volk, HD; Kox, W. Monocyte deactivation in septic patients: restoration by IFN-gamma treatment. *Nat. Med.*, 1997, 3(6), 678-681.

[20]   Reinhart, K; Karzai, W. Anti-tumor necrosis factor therapy in sepsis: update on clinical trials and lessons learned. *Crit. Care Med.*, 2001, 29(7 Suppl), S121-S125.

[21]   Walmrath, D; Grimminger, F; Seeger, W. [Severe sepsis--new therapeutic options]. *Internist (Berl)*, 2001, 42(12), 1619-1630.

[22]   Ayala, A; Herdon, CD; Lehman, DL; Ayala, CA; Chaudry, IH. Differential induction of apoptosis in lymphoid tissues during sepsis: variation in onset, frequency, and the nature of the mediators. *Blood*, 1996, 87(10), 4261-4275.

[23]   Wang, SD; Huang, KJ; Lin, YS; Lei, HY. Sepsis-induced apoptosis of the thymocytes in mice. *J. Immunol.*, 1994, 152(10), 5014-5021.

[24]   Hotchkiss, RS; Swanson, PE; Freeman, BD; Tinsley, KW; Cobb, JP; Matuschak, GM; Buchman, TG; Karl, IE. Apoptotic cell death in patients with sepsis, shock, and multiple organ dysfunction. *Crit. Care Med.*, 1999, 27(7), 1230-1251.

[25]   O'Neill, AJ; Doyle, BT; Molloy, E; Watson, C; Phelan, D; Greenan, MC; Fitzpatrick, JM; Watson, RW. Gene expression profile of inflammatory neutrophils: alterations in

the inhibitors of apoptosis proteins during spontaneous and delayed apoptosis. *Shock*, 2004 Jun, 21(6), 512 -8 2004, 21, 512-518.

[26] Sayeed, MM. Delay of neutrophil apoptosis can exacerbate inflammation in sepsis patients: cellular mechanisms. *Crit. Care Med.*, 2004 Jul, 32 (7), 1604-6 2004, 32, 1604-1606.

[27] Taneja, R; Parodo, J; Jia, SH; Kapus, A; Rotstein, OD; Marshall, JC. Delayed neutrophil apoptosis in sepsis is associated with maintenance of mitochondrial transmembrane potential and reduced caspase-9 activity. *Crit. Care Med.*, 2004 Jul, 32 (7), 1460-9 2004, 32, 1460-1469.

[28] Hotchkiss, RS; Chang, KC; Swanson, PE; Tinsley, KW; Hui, JJ; Klender, P; Xanthoudakis, S; Roy, S; Black, C; Grimm, E; Aspiotis, R; Han, Y; Nicholson, DW; Karl, IE. Caspase inhibitors improve survival in sepsis: a critical role of the lymphocyte. *Nat. Immunol.*, 2000, 1(6), 496-501.

[29] Oberholzer, C; Oberholzer, A; Clare-Salzler, M; Moldawer, LL. Apoptosis in sepsis: a new target for therapeutic exploration. *FASEB J.*, 2001, 15(6), 879-892.

[30] Nicholson, DW. From bench to clinic with apoptosis-based therapeutic agents. *Nature*, 2000, 407(6805), 810-816.

[31] Reed, JC. Apoptosis-based therapies. *Nat. Rev. Drug Discov.*, 2002, 1(2), 111-121.

[32] Kerr, JF. Shrinkage necrosis: a distinct mode of cellular death. *J. Pathol.*, 1971, 105(1), 13-20.

[33] Kerr, JF; Wyllie, AH; Currie, AR. Apoptosis: a basic biological phenomenon with wide-ranging implications in tissue kinetics. *Br. J. Cancer*, 1972, 26(4), 239-257.

[34] Hengartner, MO. The biochemistry of apoptosis. *Nature*, 2000, 407(6805), 770-776.

[35] Meier, P; Finch, A; Evan, G. Apoptosis in development. *Nature*, 2000, 407(6805), 796-801.

[36] Evan, GI; Vousden, KH. Proliferation, cell cycle and apoptosis in cancer. *Nature*, 2001, 411(6835), 342-348.

[37] Hersey, P; Zhang, XD. How melanoma cells evade trail-induced apoptosis. *Nat. Rev. Cancer*, 2001, 1(2), 142-150.

[38] Leist, M; Jaattela, M. Four deaths and a funeral: from caspases to alternative mechanisms. *Nat. Rev. Mol. Cell Biol.*, 2001, 2(8), 589-598.

[39] Wyllie, AH. Glucocorticoid-induced thymocyte apoptosis is associated with endogenous endonuclease activation. *Nature*, 1980, 284(5756), 555-556.

[40] Frasch, SC; Henson, PM; Kailey, JM; Richter, DA; Janes, MS; Fadok, VA; Bratton, DL. Regulation of phospholipid scramblase activity during apoptosis and cell activation by protein kinase Cdelta. *J. Biol. Chem.*, 2000, 275(30), 23065-23073.

[41] Anderson, HA; Maylock, CA; Williams, JA; Paweletz, CP; Shu, H; Shacter, E. Serum-derived protein S binds to phosphatidylserine and stimulates the phagocytosis of apoptotic cells. *Nat. Immunol.*, 2003, 4(1), 87-91.

[42] Jonson, DE. Noncaspase proteases in apoptosis. *Leucemia*, 2000, 14(9), 1695-1703.

[43] Mate, MJ; Ortiz-Lombardia, M; Boitel, B; Haouz, A; Tello, D; Susin, SA; Penninger, J; Kroemer, G; Alzari, PM. The crystal structure of the mouse apoptosis-inducing factor AIF. *Nat. Struct. Biol.*, 2002, 9(6), 442-446.

[44] Susin, SA; Lorenzo, HK; Zamzami, N; Marzo, I; Snow, BE; Brothers, GM; Mangion, J; Jacotot, E; Costantini, P; Loeffler, M; Larochette, N; Goodlett, DR; Aebersold, R;

Siderovski, DP; Penninger, JM; Kroemer, G. Molecular characterization of mitochondrial apoptosis-inducing factor. *Nature*, 1999, 397(6718), 441-446.

[45] Xiang, J; Chao, DT; Korsmeyer, SJ. BAX-induced cell death may not require interleukin 1 beta-converting enzyme-like proteases. *Proc. Natl. Acad. Sci. USA*, 1996, 93(25), 14559-14563.

[46] Daugas, E; Nochy, D; Ravagnan, L; Loeffler, M; Susin, SA; Zamzami, N; Kroemer, G. Apoptosis-inducing factor (AIF): a ubiquitous mitochondrial oxidoreductase involved in apoptosis. *FEBS Lett.*, 2000, 476(3), 118-123.

[47] Thornberry, NA; Lazebnik, Y. Caspases: enemies within. *Science*, 1998, 281(5381), 1312-1316.

[48] Wajant, H. The Fas signaling pathway: more than a paradigm. *Science*, 2002, 296(5573), 1635-1636.

[49] Krammer, PH. CD95's deadly mission in the immune system. *Nature*, 2000, 407(6805), 789-795.

[50] Green, DR; Ferguson, TA. The role of Fas ligand in immune privilege. *Nat. Rev. Mol. Cell Biol*, 2001, 2(12), 917-924.

[51] Khaled, AR; Durum, SK. Lymphocide: cytokines and the control of lymphoid homeostasis. *Nat. Rev. Immunol.*, 2002 Nov, 2(11), 817 -30 2002; 2, 817-830.

[52] Enari, M; Sakahira, H; Yokoyama, H; Okawa, K; Iwamatsu, A; Nagata, S. A caspase-activated DNase that degrades DNA during apoptosis, and its inhibitor ICAD. *Nature*, 1998, 391(6662), 43-50.

[53] Liu, X; Zou, H; Slaughter, C; Wang, X. DFF, a heterodimeric protein that functions downstream of caspase-3 to trigger DNA fragmentation during apoptosis. *Cell*, 1997, 89(2), 175-184.

[54] Buendia, B; Santa-Maria, A; Courvalin, JC. Caspase-dependent proteolysis of integral and peripheral proteins of nuclear membranes and nuclear pore complex proteins during apoptosis. *J. Cell Sci.*, 1999, 112 (Pt 11), 1743-1753.

[55] Kothakota, S; Azuma, T; Reinhard, C; Klippel, A; Tang, J; Chu, K; McGarry, TJ; Kirschner, MW; Koths, K; Kwiatkowski, DJ; Williams, LT. Caspase-3-generated fragment of gelsolin: effector of morphological change in apoptosis. *Science*, 1997, 278(5336), 294-298.

[56] Fadok, VA; Bratton, DL; Frasch, SC; Warner, ML; Henson, PM. The role of phosphatidylserine in recognition of apoptotic cells by phagocytes. *Cell Death Differ*, 1998, 5(7), 551-562.

[57] Martinou, JC; Green, DR. Breaking the mitochondrial barrier. *Nat Rev Mol Cell Biol*, 2001, 2(1), 63-67.

[58] Willis, SN; Adams, JM. Life in the balance: how BH3-only proteins induce apoptosis. *Curr. Opin. Cell Biol.*, 2005 Dec, 17(6), 617 -25 Epub 2005 Oct 21 2005, 17, 617-625.

[59] Cory, S; Adams, JM. The Bcl2 family: regulators of the cellular life-or-death switch. *Nat. Rev. Cancer*, 2002, 2(9), 647-656.

[60] Zamzami, N; Kroemer, G. The mitochondrion in apoptosis: how Pandora's box opens. *Nat. Rev. Mol. Cell Biol.*, 2001, 2(1), 67-71.

[61] Salvesen, GS; Duckett, CS. IAP proteins: blocking the road to death's door. *Nat. Rev. Mol. Cell Biol.*, 2002, 3(6), 401-410.

[62] Shiozaki, EN; Shi, Y. Caspases, IAPs and Smac/DIABLO: mechanisms from structural biology. *Trends Biochem. Sci.*, 2004 Sep, 29 (9), 486 -94 2004, 29, 486-494.

[63] Verhagen, AM; Ekert, PG; Pakusch, M; Silke, J; Connolly, LM; Reid, GE; Moritz, RL; Simpson, RJ; Vaux, DL. Identification of DIABLO, a mammalian protein that promotes apoptosis by binding to and antagonizing IAP proteins. *Cell*, 2000 Jul 7, 102 (1), 43 -53 2000, 102, 43-53.

[64] Chung, CS; Song, GY; Moldawer, LL; Chaudry, IH; Ayala, A. Neither Fas ligand nor endotoxin is responsible for inducible peritoneal phagocyte apoptosis during sepsis/peritonitis. *J. Surg. Res.*, 2000, 91(2), 147-153.

[65] Ayala, A; Lomas, JL; Grutkoski, PS; Chung, CS. Pathological aspects of apoptosis in severe sepsis and shock? *Int. J. Biochem. Cell Biol.*, 2003, 35(1), 7-15.

[66] Ayala, A; Chung, CS; Lomas, JL; Song, GY; Doughty, LA; Gregory, SH; Cioffi, WG; LeBlanc, BW; Reichner, J; Simms, HH; Grutkoski, PS. Shock-induced neutrophil mediated priming for acute lung injury in mice: divergent effects of TLR-4 and TLR-4/FasL deficiency. *Am. J. Pathol.*, 2002, 161(6), 2283-2294.

[67] Chung, CS; Yang, S; Song, GY; Lomas, J; Wang, P; Simms, HH; Chaudry, IH; Ayala, A. Inhibition of Fas signaling prevents hepatic injury and improves organ blood flow during sepsis. *Surgery*, 2001, 130(2), 339-345.

[68] Chung, CS; Wang, W; Chaudry, IH; Ayala, A. Increased apoptosis in lamina propria B cells during polymicrobial sepsis is FasL but not endotoxin mediated. *Am. J. Physiol. Gastrointest Liver Physiol.*, 2001, 280(5), G812-G818.

[69] Ayala, A; Chung, CS; Xu, YX; Evans, TA; Redmond, KM; Chaudry, IH. Increased inducible apoptosis in CD4+ T lymphocytes during polymicrobial sepsis is mediated by Fas ligand and not endotoxin. *Immunology*, 1999, 97(1), 45-55.

[70] Wesche-Soldato, DE; Chung, CS; Lomas-Neira, J; Doughty, LA; Gregory, SH; Ayala, A. In vivo delivery of caspase-8 or Fas siRNA improves the survival of septic mice. *Blood*, 2005 Oct 1, 106 (7), 2295 -301 Epub 2005 Jun 7 2005, 106, 2295-2301.

[71] Cobb, JP; Laramie, JM; Stormo, GD; Morrissey, JJ; Shannon, WD; Qiu, Y; Karl, IE; Buchman, TG; Hotchkiss, RS. Sepsis gene expression profiling: murine splenic compared with hepatic responses determined by using complementary DNA microarrays. *Crit. Care Med.*, 2002, 30(12), 2711-2721.

[72] Hotchkiss, RS; Dunne, WM; Swanson, PE; Davis, CG; Tinsley, KW; Chang, KC; Buchman, TG; Karl, IE. Role of apoptosis in Pseudomonas aeruginosa pneumonia. *Science*, 2001, 294(5548), 1783.

[73] Freeman, BD; Reaume, AG; Swanson, PE; Epstein, CJ; Carlson, EJ; Buchman, TG; Karl, IE; Hotchkiss, RS. Role of CuZn superoxide dismutase in regulating lymphocyte apoptosis during sepsis. *Crit. Care Med.*, 2000, 28(6), 1701-1708.

[74] Hotchkiss, RS; Tinsley, KW; Hui, JJ; Chang, KC; Swanson, PE; Drewry, AM; Buchman, TG; Karl, IE. p53-dependent and -independent pathways of apoptotic cell death in sepsis. *J Immunol*, 2000, 164(7), 3675-3680.

[75] Tinsley, KW; Cheng, SL; Buchman, TG; Chang, KC; Hui, JJ; Swanson, PE; Karl, IE; Hotchkiss, RS. Caspases -2, -3, -6, and -9, but not caspase-1, are activated in sepsis-induced thymocyte apoptosis. *Shock*, 2000, 13(1), 1-7.

[76] Hotchkiss, RS; Tinsley, KW; Swanson, PE; Chang, KC; Cobb, JP; Buchman, TG; Korsmeyer, SJ; Karl, IE. Prevention of lymphocyte cell death in sepsis improves survival in mice. *Proc. Natl. Acad. Sci. USA*, 1999, 96(25), 14541-14546.

[77] Hotchkiss, RS; Swanson, PE; Knudson, CM; Chang, KC; Cobb, JP; Osborne, DF; Zollner, KM; Buchman, TG; Korsmeyer, SJ; Karl, IE. Overexpression of Bcl-2 in

transgenic mice decreases apoptosis and improves survival in sepsis. *J. Immunol.*, 1999, 162(7), 4148-4156.

[78] Hiramatsu, M; Hotchkiss, RS; Karl, IE; Buchman, TG. Cecal ligation and puncture (CLP) induces apoptosis in thymus, spleen, lung, and gut by an endotoxin and TNF-independent pathway. *Shock*, 1997, 7(4), 247-253.

[79] Bommhardt, U; Chang, KC; Swanson, PE; Wagner, TH; Tinsley, KW; Karl, IE; Hotchkiss, RS. Akt decreases lymphocyte apoptosis and improves survival in sepsis. *J. Immunol.*, 2004, 172(12), 7583-7591.

[80] Schroeder, S; Lindemann, C; Decker, D; Klaschik, S; Hering, R; Putensen, C; Hoeft, A; von Ruecker, A; Stuber, F. Increased susceptibility to apoptosis in circulating lymphocytes of critically ill patients. *Langenbecks Arch. Surg.*, 2001, 386(1), 42-46.

[81] Papathanassoglou, ED; Moynihan, JA; McDermott, MP; Ackerman, MH. Expression of Fas (CD95) and Fas ligand on peripheral blood mononuclear cells in critical illness and association with multiorgan dysfunction severity and survival. *Crit. Care Med.*, 2001, 29(4), 709-718.

[82] Hotchkiss, RS; Tinsley, KW; Swanson, PE; Grayson, MH; Osborne, DF; Wagner, TH; Cobb, JP; Coopersmith, C; Karl, IE. Depletion of dendritic cells, but not macrophages, in patients with sepsis. *J. Immunol.*, 2002, 168(5), 2493-2500.

[83] Hotchkiss, RS; Tinsley, KW; Swanson, PE; Schmieg, RE; Jr., Hui, JJ; Chang, KC; Osborne, DF; Freeman, BD; Cobb, JP; Buchman, TG; Karl, IE. Sepsis-induced apoptosis causes progressive profound depletion of B and CD4+ T lymphocytes in humans. *J. Immunol.*, 2001, 166(11), 6952-6963.

[84] Hotchkiss, RS; Osmon, SB; Chang, KC; Wagner, TH; Coopersmith, CM; Karl, IE. Accelerated lymphocyte death in sepsis occurs by both the death receptor and mitochondrial pathways. *J. Immunol.*, 2005 Apr 15, 174 (8), 5110-8 2005, 174, 5110-5118.

[85] Nathan, C. Points of control in inflammation. *Nature*, 2002, 420(6917), 846-852.

[86] Henriksson, CE; Hellum, M; Landsverk, KS; Klingenberg, O; Joo, GB; Kierulf, P. Flow cytometry-sorted non-viable endotoxin-treated human monocytes are strongly procoagulant. *Thromb. Haemost*, 2006 Jul, 96 (1), 29 -37 2006, 96, 29-37.

[87] Hotchkiss, RS; Chang, KC; Grayson, MH; Tinsley, KW; Dunne, BS; Davis, CG; Osborne, DF; Karl, IE. Adoptive transfer of apoptotic splenocytes worsens survival, whereas adoptive transfer of necrotic splenocytes improves survival in sepsis. *Proc. Natl. Acad. Sci. USA*, 2003 May 27, 100 (11), 6724 -9 Epub 2003 May 7 2003, 100, 6724-6729.

[88] Venet, F; Pachot, A; Debard, AL; Bohe, J; Bienvenu, J; Lepape, A; Monneret, G. Increased percentage of CD4+CD25+ regulatory T cells during septic shock is due to the decrease of CD4+CD25- lymphocytes. *Crit. Care Med.*, 2004 Nov, 32 (11), 2329-31 2004, 32, 2329-2331.

[89] Carson, WE, Yu, H; Dierksheide, J; Pfeffer, K; Bouchard, P; Clark, R; Durbin, J; Baldwin, AS; Peschon, J; Johnson, PR; Ku, G; Baumann, H; Caligiuri, MA. A fatal cytokine-induced systemic inflammatory response reveals a critical role for NK cells. *J. Immunol.*, 1999, 162, 4943-4951.

[90] Chung, CS; Watkins, L; Funches, A; Lomas-Neira, J; Cioffi, WG; Ayala, A. DEFICIENCY OF {gamma}{delta} T-Lymphocytes Contributes To Mortality And

Immunosuppression In Sepsis. *Am. J. Physiol. Regul. Integr. Comp. Physiol.*, 2006 Jun 22, 2006.

[91] Adrie, C; Bachelet, M; Vayssier-Taussat, M; Russo-Marie, F; Bouchaert, I; Adib-Conquy, M; Cavaillon, JM; Pinsky, MR; Dhainaut, JF; Polla, BS. Mitochondrial membrane potential and apoptosis peripheral blood monocytes in severe human sepsis. *Am. J. Respir. Crit. Care Med.*, 2001, 164(3), 389-395.

[92] Tinsley, KW; Grayson, MH; Swanson, PE; Drewry, AM; Chang, KC; Karl, IE; Hotchkiss, RS. Sepsis induces apoptosis and profound depletion of splenic interdigitating and follicular dendritic cells. *J. Immunol.*, 2003, 171(2), 909-914.

[93] Efron, PA; Martins, A; Minnich, D; Tinsley, K; Ungaro, R; Bahjat, FR; Hotchkiss, R; Clare-Salzler, M; Moldawer, LL. Characterization of the systemic loss of dendritic cells in murine lymph nodes during polymicrobial sepsis. *J. Immunol.*, 2004 Sep 1, 173 (5), 3035 -43 2004, 173, 3035-3043.

[94] Riedemann, NC; Guo, RF; Laudes, IJ; Keller, K; Sarma, VJ; Padgaonkar, V; Zetoune, FS; Ward, PA. C5a receptor and thymocyte apoptosis in sepsis. *FASEB J.*, 2002, 16(8), 887-888.

[95] Baker, CC; Chaudry, IH; Gaines, HO; Baue, AE. Evaluation of factors affecting mortality rate after sepsis in a murine cecal ligation and puncture model. *Surgery*, 1983, 94(2), 331-335.

[96] Ayala, A; Herdon, CD; Lehman, DL; DeMaso, CM; Ayala, CA; Chaudry, IH. The induction of accelerated thymic programmed cell death during polymicrobial sepsis: control by corticosteroids but not tumor necrosis factor. *Shock*, 1995, 3(4), 259-267.

[97] Miura, M; Zhu, H; Rotello, R; Hartwieg, EA; Yuan, J. Induction of apoptosis in fibroblasts by IL-1 beta-converting enzyme, a mammalian homolog of the C. elegans cell death gene ced-3. *Cell*, 1993, 75(4), 653-660.

[98] Bump, NJ; Hackett, M; Hugunin, M; Seshagiri, S; Brady, K; Chen, P; Ferenz, C; Franklin, S; Ghayur, T; Li, P. Inhibition of ICE family proteases by baculovirus antiapoptotic protein p35. *Science*, 1995, 269(5232), 1885-1888.

[99] Kang, SJ; Wang, S; Kuida, K; Yuan, J. Distinct downstream pathways of caspase-11 in regulating apoptosis and cytokine maturation during septic shock response. *Cell Death Differ*, 2002 Oct, 9 (10), 1115 -25 2002, 9, 1115-1125.

[100] Saleh, M; Mathison, JC; Wolinski, MK; Bensinger, SJ; Fitzgerald, P; Droin, N; Ulevitch, RJ; Green, DR; Nicholson, DW. Enhanced bacterial clearance and sepsis resistance in caspase-12-deficient mice. *Nature*, 2006 Apr 20, 440 (7087), 1064-8 2006; 440, 1064-1068.

[101] Ayala, A; Lomas, JL; Grutkoski, PS; Chung, S. Fas-ligand mediated apoptosis in severe sepsis and shock. *Scand. J. Infect. Dis.*, 2003, 35 (9), 593 -600 2003, 35, 593-600.

[102] Chung, CS; Song, GY; Lomas, J; Simms, HH; Chaudry, IH; Ayala, A. Inhibition of Fas/Fas ligand signaling improves septic survival: differential effects on macrophage apoptotic and functional capacity. *J. Leukoc. Biol.*, 2003 Sep; 74 (3), 344-51 2003, 74, 344-351.

[103] Ferri, KF; Kroemer, G. Organelle-specific initiation of cell death pathways. *Nat. Cell Biol.*, 2001 Nov, 3(11), E255-63 2001, 3, E255-E263.

[104] Hotchkiss, RS; McConnell, KW; Bullok, K; Davis, CG; Chang, KC; Schwulst, SJ; Dunne, JC; Dietz, GP; Bahr, M; McDunn, JE; Karl, IE; Wagner, TH; Cobb, JP; Coopersmith, CM; Piwnica-Worms, D. TAT-BH4 and TAT-Bcl-xL peptides protect

against sepsis-induced lymphocyte apoptosis in vivo. *J Immunol*, 2006 May 1, 176 (9), 5471-7 2006, 176, 5471-5477.

[105] Welte, K; Zeidler, C; Dale, DC. Severe congenital neutropenia. *Semin. Hematol.*, 2006 Jul, 43 (3), 189-95 2006, 43, 189-195.

[106] Kollner, I; Sodeik, B; Schreek, S; Heyn, H; von Neuhoff, N; Germeshausen, M; Zeidler, C; Kruger, M; Schlegelberger, B; Welte, K; Beger, C. Mutations in neutrophil elastase causing congenital neutropenia lead to cytoplasmic protein accumulation and induction of the unfolded protein response. *Blood*, 2006 Jul. 15, 108 (2), 493-500 Epub 2006 Mar 21 2006, 108, 493-500.

[107] Dale, DC; Person, RE; Bolyard, AA; Aprikyan, AG; Bos, C; Bonilla, MA; Boxer, LA; Kannourakis, G; Zeidler, C; Welte, K; Benson, KF; Horwitz, M. Mutations in the gene encoding neutrophil elastase in congenital and cyclic neutropenia. *Blood*, 2000 Oct 1, 96 (7), 2317-22 2000, 96, 2317-2322.

[108] Bonilla, MA; Gillio, AP; Ruggeiro, M; Kernan, NA; Brochstein, JA; Abboud, M; Fumagalli, L; Vincent, M; Gabrilove, JL; Welte, K. Effects of recombinant human granulocyte colony-stimulating factor on neutropenia in patients with congenital agranulocytosis. *N. Engl. J. Med.*, 1989, 320, 1574-1580.

[109] Welte, K; Bonilla, MA; Gillio, AP; Boone, TC; Potter, GK; Gabrilove, JL; Moore, MA; O'Reilly, RJ; Souza, LM. Recombinant human granulocyte colony-stimulating factor. Effects on hematopoiesis in normal and cyclophosphamide-treated primates. *J. Exp. Med.*, 1987, 165, 941-948.

[110] Matute-Bello, G; Liles, WC; Radella, F; Steinberg, KP; Ruzinski, JT; Jonas, M; Chi, EY; Hudson, LD; Martin, TR. Neutrophil apoptosis in the acute respiratory distress syndrome. *Am. J. Respir. Crit. Care Med.*, 1997, 156, 1969-1977.

[111] Brown, KA; Brain, SD; Pearson, JD; Edgeworth, JD; Lewis, SM; Treacher, DF. Neutrophils in development of multiple organ failure in sepsis. *Lancet*, 2006 Jul 8, 368 (9530), 157-69 2006, 368, 157-169.

[112] Matute-Bello, G; Martin, TR. Science review: apoptosis in acute lung injury. *Crit. Care*, 2003 Oct, 7 (5), 355-8 Epub 2003 Apr 4 2003, 7, 355-358.

[113] Keel, M; Ungethum, U; Steckholzer, U; Niederer, E; Hartung, T; Trentz, O; Ertel, W. Interleukin-10 counterregulates proinflammatory cytokine-induced inhibition of neutrophil apoptosis during severe sepsis. *Blood*, 1997, 90, 3356-3363.

[114] Aranow, JS; Fink, MP. Determinants of intestinal barrier failure in critical illness. *Br. J. Anaesth.*, 1996, 77(1), 71-81.

[115] Deitch, EA; Bridges, W; Baker, J; Ma, JW; Ma, L; Grisham, MB; Granger, DN; Specian, RD; Berg, R. Hemorrhagic shock-induced bacterial translocation is reduced by xanthine oxidase inhibition or inactivation. *Surgery*, 1988, 104(2), 191-198.

[116] Maloney, JP; Halbower, AC; Fouty, BF; Fagan, KA; Balasubramaniam, V; Pike, AW; Fennessey, PV; Moss, M. Systemic absorption of food dye in patients with sepsis. *N. Engl. J. Med.*, 2000, 343(14), 1047-1048.

[117] Hotchkiss, RS; Swanson, PE; Cobb, JP; Jacobson, A; Buchman, TG; Karl, IE. Apoptosis in lymphoid and parenchymal cells during sepsis: findings in normal and T- and B-cell-deficient mice. *Crit. Care Med.*, 1997, 25(8), 1298-1307.

[118] Coopersmith, CM; Chang, KC; Swanson, PE; Tinsley, KW; Stromberg, PE; Buchman, TG; Karl, IE; Hotchkiss, RS. Overexpression of Bcl-2 in the intestinal epithelium improves survival in septic mice. *Crit. Care Med.*, 2002, 30(1), 195-201.

[119] Beranek, JT. Cardiomyocyte apoptosis contributes to the pathology of the septic shock heart. *Intensive Care Med.*, 2002 Feb, 28 (2), 218, author reply 219 Epub 2002 Jan 12 2002, 28, 218.

[120] Crouser, ED. Redefining the roles of apoptosis pathways during sepsis. *Crit Care Med*, 2005 Mar, 33 (3), 670 -2 2005, 33, 670-672.

[121] Lancel, S; Joulin, O; Favory, R; Goossens, JF; Kluza, J; Chopin, C; Formstecher, P; Marchetti, P; Neviere, R. Ventricular myocyte caspases are directly responsible for endotoxin-induced cardiac dysfunction. *Circulation*, 2005 May 24, 111 (20), 2596 -604 Epub 2005 May 16 2005, 111, 2596-2604.

[122] Lancel, S; Petillot, P; Favory, R; Stebach, N; Lahorte, C; Danze, PM; Vallet, B; Marchetti, P; Neviere, R. Expression of apoptosis regulatory factors during myocardial dysfunction in endotoxemic rats. *Crit. Care Med.*, 2005 Mar, 33 (3), 492-6 2005, 33, 492-496.

[123] Crouser, ED. Is cell death a prerequisite for cardiac dysfunction during sepsis? *Crit. Care Med.*, 2005 May, 33 (5), 1160-2 2005, 33, 1160-1162.

[124] Carlson, DL; Willis, MS; White, DJ; Horton, JW; Giroir, BP. Tumor necrosis factor-alpha-induced caspase activation mediates endotoxin-related cardiac dysfunction. *Crit. Care Med.*, 2005 May, 33 (5), 1021-8 2005, 33, 1021-1028.

[125] Martin, TR; Nakamura, M; Matute-Bello, G. The role of apoptosis in acute lung injury. *Crit. Care Med.*, 2003 Apr, 31 (4 Suppl), S184-8 2003, 31, S184-S188.

[126] Matute-Bello, G; Frevert, CW; Liles, WC; Nakamura, M; Ruzinski, JT; Ballman, K; Wong, VA; Vathanaprida, C; Martin, TR. Fas/Fas ligand system mediates epithelial injury, but not pulmonary host defenses, in response to inhaled bacteria. *Infect. Immun.*, 2001 Sep, 69 (9), 5768-76 2001, 69, 5768-5776.

[127] Matute-Bello, G; Winn, RK; Jonas, M; Chi, EY; Martin, TR; Liles, WC. Fas (CD95) induces alveolar epithelial cell apoptosis in vivo: implications for acute pulmonary inflammation. *Am. J. Pathol.*, 2001 Jan, 158 (1), 153-61 2001, 158, 153-161.

[128] Hotchkiss, RS; Tinsley, KW; Swanson, PE; Karl, IE. Endothelial cell apoptosis in sepsis. *Crit. Care Med.*, 2002, 30(5 Suppl), S225-S228.

[129] Zeerleder, S; Zwart, B; Wuillemin, WA; Aarden, LA; Groeneveld, AB; Caliezi, C; van Nieuwenhuijze, AE; van Mierlo, GJ; Eerenberg, AJ; Lammle, B; Hack, CE. Elevated nucleosome levels in systemic inflammation and sepsis. *Crit. Care Med.*, 2003 Jul, 31 (7), 1947 -51 2003, 31, 1947-1951.

[130] Bilbault, P; Lavaux, T; Lahlou, A; Uring-Lambert, B; Gaub, MP; Ratomponirina, C; Meyer, N; Oudet, P; Schneider, F. Transient Bcl-2 gene down-expression in circulating mononuclear cells of severe sepsis patients who died despite appropriate intensive care. *Intensive Care Med.*, 2004 Mar, 30 (3), 408 -15 Epub 2004 Jan 13 2004, 30, 408-415.

[131] Roth, G; Moser, B; Krenn, C; Brunner, M; Haisjackl, M; Almer, G; Gerlitz, S; Wolner, E; Boltz-Nitulescu, G; Ankersmit, HJ. Susceptibility to programmed cell death in T-lymphocytes from septic patients: a mechanism for lymphopenia and Th2 predominance. *Biochem. Biophys Res. Commun.*, 2003 Sep 5, 308 (4), 840-6 2003, 308, 840-846.

[132] Doughty, L; Clark, RS; Kaplan, SS; Sasser, H; Carcillo, J. sFas and sFas ligand and pediatric sepsis-induced multiple organ failure syndrome. *Pediatr. Res.*, 2002 Dec, 52 (6), 922-7 2002, 52, 922-927.

[133] Papathanassoglou, ED; Moynihan, JA; Vermillion, DL; McDermott, MP; Ackerman, MH. Soluble fas levels correlate with multiple organ dysfunction severity, survival and nitrate levels, but not with cellular apoptotic markers in critically ill patients. *Shock* 2000 Aug, 14(2), 107-12 2000, 14, 107-112.

[134] Torre, D; Tambini, R; Manfredi, M; Mangani, V; Livi, P; Maldifassi, V; Campi, P; Speranza, F. Circulating levels of FAS/APO-1 in patients with the systemic inflammatory response syndrome. *Diagn. Microbiol. Infect. Dis.*, 2003 Apr, 45 (4), 233-6 2003, 45, 233-236.

[135] De, F; I, Fernandez-Somoza, M; Essenfeld-Sekler, E; Cardier, JE. Serum levels of the apoptosis-associated molecules, tumor necrosis factor-alpha/tumor necrosis factor type-I receptor and Fas/FasL, in sepsis. *Chest*, 2004 Jun, 125 (6), 2238-46 2004, 125, 2238-2246.

[136] Marsik, C; Halama, T; Cardona, F; Wlassits, W; Mayr, F; Pleiner, J; Jilma, B. Regulation of Fas (APO-1, CD95) and Fas ligand expression in leukocytes during systemic inflammation in humans. *Shock*, 2003 Dec, 20 (6), 493-6 2003, 20, 493-496.

[137] Marsik, C; Halama, T; Cardona, F; Wlassits, W; Mayr, F; Pleiner, J; Jilma, B. Regulation of Fas (APO-1, CD95) and Fas ligand expression in leukocytes during systemic inflammation in humans. *Shock*, 2003 Dec, 20 (6), 493-6 2003, 20, 493-496.

[138] Flohe, SB; Agrawal, H; Schmitz, D; Gertz, M; Flohe, S; Schade, FU. Dendritic cells during polymicrobial sepsis rapidly mature but fail to initiate a protective Th1-type immune response. *J. Leukoc. Biol.*, 2006 Mar, 79 (3), 473-81 Epub 2005 Dec 2006, 79, 473-481.

[139] Riedemann, NC; Guo, RF; Ward, PA. The enigma of sepsis. *J. Clin. Invest.*, 2003, 112(4), 460-467.

[140] Riedemann, NC; Guo, RF; Ward, PA. Novel strategies for the treatment of sepsis. *Nat. Med.*, 2003 May, 9 (5), 517-24 2003, 9, 517-524.

[141] Oberholzer, A; Oberholzer, C; Minter, RM; Moldawer, LL. Considering immunomodulatory therapies in the septic patient: should apoptosis be a potential therapeutic target? *Immunol Lett.*, 2001, 75(3), 221-224.

In: Sepsis: Symptoms, Diagnosis and Treatment
Editor: Joseph R. Brown, pp. 129-151

ISBN: 978-1-60876-609-3
© 2010 Nova Science Publishers, Inc.

Chapter 7

MANAGEMENT OF SEPSIS

Jochanan E. Naschitz and Alona Paz

Technion-Israel Institute of Technology, Haifa, Israel

Sepsis is the term used to describe the body's systemic responses to infection. A consensus committee of American experts in 1992 defined sepsis as a systemic inflammatory response syndrome due to presumed or confirmed infection. Nonspecific symptoms such as tachycardia, leukocytosis and fever may be inflammatory in nature; when occurring in concert they constitute the 'systemic inflammatory response syndrome' (SIRS). SIRS occurring in a patient with proven or suspected infection is called 'sepsis' [1]. A review of the National Hospital Discharge Survey (U.S.A) data found that the incidence of sepsis increased by almost fourfold during the interval from 1979 to 2000, to 240 cases per 100,000 population per year [2].

Sepsis causes considerable morbidity, cost, health care utilization and mortality. Hospital mortality for sepsis patients ranges from 18% to 30%, depending on the series. While the mortality rate has decreased over the past 20 years, an increase in the number of sepsis cases has resulted in a tripling of the number of sepsis-related deaths [3]. There is a growing awareness of the need for an organized approach to caring for patients affected by sepsis. An early diagnosis of sepsis, prior to the onset of clinical decline, allows for prompt antibiotic administration and goal-directed resuscitation. The time to initiate therapy is thought to be crucial and the major determining factor for surviving sepsis [4,5], similar to the critical time-limit for early interventions in management of acute myocardial infarction and ischemic stroke.

Elderly patients are at increased risk to develop sepsis. In fact, age greater than 65 years is associated with a 13.1 times increased risk to contract sepsis vs age less than 65 years [6]. Hence, appropriate care for sepsis is a major issue in the acute geriatric ward. The spread of multidrug-resistant Gram-negative and Gram-positive organisms in geriatric wards implies the need to delay development of antibiotic resistance. To this aim, choosing the right drugs and dosing regimens, monitoring antibiotics use and avoidance of their overuse are important measures [7,8].

This chapter will center on the diagnosis and management of sepsis in the geriatric ward and on infection containment. Preference will be given to problems faced more recently by the authors.

I. BASICS

For sepsis to occur, a large bacterial inoculum must break the host's defenses [3]. Nearly all bacteria are capable of causing sepsis, at least in immuno-compromised patients. Many infections arise from the patient's own bacterial flora. *Staphylococcus epidermidis* normally colonizes the human skin, but when it invades the bloodstream, it can cause septicemia, endocarditis, or infections of prosthetic joints. *Staphylococcus aureus* colonizes the skin and mucosal surfaces in the nose in 30% of the population. When it extends to other sites, staphylococcus aureus can cause skin abscesses, arthritis, endocarditis and necrotizing pneumonia. When bacteria from the oral cavity are aspirated to the lungs pneumonia can evolve. *Escherichia coli,* which is a normal inhabitant of the gut, may enter the blood stream and cause a variety of infections. Bacteria are often considered the sole causative agents of sepsis, but any microorganism can cause sepsis, including fungi, parasites, and viruses [3].

The interaction of microbiological products with a susceptible host induces a cascade of immunomodulatory mediators which are largely responsible for the clinical symptoms and signs of sepsis. So, sepsis is the systemic inflammatory response syndrome secondary to an infection, a dynamic process caused by imbalance in the 'inflammatory network' [9]. The major pathways involved in sepsis include the innate immune response, inflammatory cascades, procoagulant and antifibrinolytic pathways, alterations in cellular metabolism and signaling, and an acquired immune dysfunction [3]. A detailed description of the mechanisms operative in sepsis is beyond the aim of the present discussion, and can be found in recently published reviews [10-12].

Aging is accompanied by the decline in cell-mediated and humoral immune functions, contributing to the enhanced susceptibility to infection. In the elderly, cytokine and chemokine signaling networks are altered with a predominant type 2 cytokine response over type 1 cytokine response; induction of proinflammatory cytokines after septic stimuli is inadequately controlled by anti-inflammatory mechanisms. The pathophysiologic cascades operative in sepsis, when insufficiently countered by homeostatic defenses, may render elderly patients at increased risk for major organ dysfunction, shock and death [13].

The clinical manifestations of sepsis comprise a spectrum that ranges from minor signs and symptoms to organ dysfunction and shock [14]. At first presentation, symptoms of sepsis may be atypical, sometimes making early diagnosis difficult. Altered mental status may be the sole presenting sign of sepsis in elderly subjects. Atypical presentations, such as the absence of fever, tachycardia or leukocytosis, are more prevalent in the older age groups. This is illustrated in a notable study comparing the manifestations of bloodstream infections at different ages [15]. The oldest patients (≥85 years old) and elderly patients (65-84 years old) had more often atypical manifestations, more frequent organ failure and a worse prognosis than younger adults (18-64 years old). Elderly patients had significantly less tachycardia, more often acute respiratory failure and renal failure. Sepsis in the oldest old patients occurred more without fever and leukocytosis, while the oldest old developed more often respiratory failure, acute renal failure, septic shock, and altered mental status. Urinary tract infections were the main source of blood stream infections for both the elderly and oldest old. The oldest old had significantly more pneumonia than the elderly or younger adults. The oldest old patients had a significantly higher frequency of polymicrobial bacteremia. The three most common bacteria across age classes were Escherichia coli, Klebsiella pneumoniae and Staphylococcus aureus [15]. In another study, oldest old bacteremic patients had higher percentage of infections with Gram-negative organisms and Staphylococcus aureus, empirical antibiotic treatment was more often inappropriate, and bacteremia-related mortality was greater [16].

A favorable outcome of sepsis depends on early and aggressive treatment. Implementation of a comprehensive sepsis treatment protocol is feasible and is associated with changes in therapies such as administration of antibiotics, delivery of intravenous fluids, and use of vasopressor in the first 6 hours after onset of symptoms [4,5].

II. SEPSIS MANAGEMENT ROUTINE

A routine should be followed to optimize the management of sepsis: blood and urine cultures should be taken; imaging studies be performed promptly to confirm the potential source of infection; empirical treatment with a broad-spectrum antibiotic be immediately started; subtle signs of organ hypoperfusion should be pursued and corrected; after results of microbiology cultures are awailable, the antibiotic coverage needs to be narrowed as appropriate [17,18].

Collection of Specimens

Often physicians are unfamiliar with guidelines for specimen collection and transport; emphasis on technical details on this subject is desirable [19]. Collection of specimens for culture of specific microorganisms should start before the administration of chemotherapeutic agents so that the recovery of microorganisms will not be compromised. Careful collection may prevent the specimen's contamination with normal flora. For instance, blood cultures should always be taken with gloves, the venipuncture site should be prepared either with povidone-iodine, or 70% alcohol; both are applied in a circular fashion to the puncture site. Then, 10 to 20 mL of blood are drawn and injected into the blood culture bottles. These are to be transported ASAP to the microbiology laboratory to start incubation. Upon suspicion of infection of a central venous catheter, the catheter should be removed aseptically and a 4 cm segment or longer cut from the tip should be placed in a sterile container. For urine cultures, a midstream specimen should be properly collected. Straight catheter collection provides proper specimen without or less contamination. Urine cultures may either be transported promptly to the laboratory or kept refrigerated. In distinction from intravenous catheters, urinary catheters are not acceptable for culture [19].

Antibiotic Treatment for Sepsis

The choice of empiric antibiotics depends on the clinical syndrome, underlying disease, susceptibility patterns of pathogens in the community and in the hospital, susceptibility of pathogens that previously have been shown to colonize or infect the patient, as well as the patient's drug intolerances [18]. Because patients with severe sepsis or septic shock have little margin for error in the choice of therapy, the initial selection of antimicrobial therapy should be wide-ranging to cover all likely pathogens. Failure to initiate appropriate therapy correlates with increased morbidity and mortality [20-22].

Empirical antimicrobial therapy depends upon localizing the site of infection to a particular organ, which indicates the probable pathogenic flora in the septic process and is the basis for the selection of appropriate empiric antimicrobial therapy [23]. The most common conditions associated with sepsis are urinary infections, pulmonaty, hepatobiliary, colon and pelvic infections, central venous catheter infections and intravascular infections. The possibility of nosocomial infection with multidrug resistant pathogens is a major consideration [24]. Recently used antibiotics should generally be avoided. *Monotherapy* is preferred to polypharmacy, which increases costs, potential for side effects and for drug–drug interactions. Patients should receive a full loading dose of each antimicrobial, but in taking account that patients with sepsis or septic shock often have abnormal renal or hepatic function and may have abnormal volumes of distribution due to aggressive fluid resuscitation. *Combination therapy* is recommended for patients with known or suspected pseudomonas or enterococcus as a cause of severe sepsis; also combination empirical therapy is recommended for neutropenic patients with severe sepsis. When used empirically in patients with severe sepsis, combination therapy should not be administered for longer than 3–5 days [23].

When results of microbiology become available, antibiotic therapy is reassessed to narrow the coverage [18]. It may become apparent that none of the empirical drugs that have been administered offer optimal therapy; there may be another drug proven to produce superior clinical outcome that should therefore replace empirical agents. Narrowing the spectrum of antibiotic coverage and reducing the duration of antibiotic therapy reduces the likelihood that the patient will develop superinfection with pathogenic or resistant organisms, such as Candida species, Clostridium difficile, or vancomycin-resistant Enterococcus faecium. However, the wish for minimizing superinfections should not take priority over the need to give the patient an adequate time of treatment to cure the infection which caused the severe sepsis or septic shock [18]. De-escalation is not necessary if initial monotherapy was suitable [23]. Drug serum concentration monitoring can be useful for those drugs that can be measured promptly [18].

Local unit specific antimicrobial sensitivity data are important in selecting empiric therapy and institutional practices for management of sepsis have been proposed. Illustrative is the Winthrop-University Hospital protocol [23], based on prevalence of pathogens and their sensitivities to antibiotics in the USA. Accordingly, if the probable source of infection is the lower gastrointestinal tract or pelvis, meropenem treatment is initiated empirically giving coverage to possible B. fragilis infection; for suspected aerobic Gram negative bacteria tigecycline is started; if the probable source of infection is the genitourinary tract, piperacillin-tazobactam is recommended directed against aerobic Gram negative bacteria or meropenem against Enterococcus faecalis; if the probable source of infection is a central venous line and the probable pathogen is S. aureus, empirical treatment with meropenem is started; in institutions where central line infections due to MRSA are more prevalent vancomycin, daptomycin, or linezolid is recommended; for aerobic Gram negative bacteria tigercycline is prescribed; for nosocomial pneumonia meropenem treatment is started to give broad spectrum coverage inclusive for Pseudomonas aeruginosa, or cefepime for possible aerobic Gram negative bacteria [23].

In other countries or other hospitals with different prevalence of pathogens and different antibiotic sensitivities, different institutional protocols for initiation of empirical antibiotic treatment of sepsis may be useful. Emphasis is given to unit specific choces of empiric antibiotic treatment [3,23,25-27].

General Supportive Measures in the Treatment of Sepsis

Circulatory impairment in sepsis is the consequence of vasodilatation, capillary leak, and reduced myocardial contractility. For volume resuscitation crystalloids and colloids are used, but it remains unresolved whether colloids have an advantage over intravenous crystalloids [17]. Concerning administration of human albumin for volume resuscitation, studies showed that intravenous albumin treatment was associated with a 6% excess mortality or no benefit in outcome [28,29]. Circulatory compromise should be corrected early and effectively, but achievement of this aim is hindered by inaccuracy of the methods which estimate the effective intravascular volume. For guidance most physicians will rely on clinical endpoints such as sustained increase in blood pressure, increase in central venous pressure, decrease in heart rate, increased urine output, improovement of base deficit and blood lactate concentration [17]. However, global hemodynamic parameters do not provide adequate information on tissue perfusion [30]. Furthermore, mixed venous oxygen saturation and blood lactate – the global 'downstream' markers of impaired tissue perfusion - are insensitive indicators of tissue hypoxia [31]. Other indicators of optimal fluid resuscitations are needed. Thoracic impedance monitoring, which allows for early diagnosis of pulmonary congestion and can predict decompensation in patients with heart failure [32,33], has not been sufficiently explored for monitoring fluid resuscitation. Transesophageal Doppler echocardiography [34], as well as pulse contour analysis, provides information on the effect of fluid loading on cardiac output [35]; their value in the management of fluid resuscitation needs to be confirmed by further studies. Monitoring the pulmonary capillary wedge pressure showed no benefit in patients with severe sepsis [17]. In distinction to the shortages of the various methods mentioned above, assessment of the peripheral perfusion allows for very early diagnosis of hypoperfusion in the microcirculation and may become the preferred technique in the setting of intensive care units [28]. Monitoring the course of sepsis by observing the microcirculation is discussed in more detail in the chapter 'Normotensive Shock'.

Administration of catecholamines is needed when adequate tissue perfusion cannot be achieved by intravenous fluids. Either noradrenaline or dopamine is recommended as first line agent. The quality of evidence is poor for the choice of particular vasopressor agents to support the circulation in sepsis [17]. Dopamine exhibits a graded pharmacological response, with a dose-dependent predominant activation of dopaminergic receptors, β-receptors, and ά-receptors. Generally, at doses <3 μg/ kg/min, dopamine activates dopamine A1 receptors, which dilate the renal arteries and other vascular beds, including mesenteric, coronary, and cerebral vascular beds. Stimulation of dopamine A2 receptors by dopamine leads to inhibition of norepinephrine release from sympathetic nerve endings. Activation of dopamine A1 and A2 receptors also results in a decline in systemic vascular resistance and an increase in renal blood flow [36]. Low-dose dopamine, that has been much used in the past mainly because it increases the splanchnic blood flow, has been proscribed in recent years. Low-dose dopamine does not improve hepatic function, it inhibits gut motility, mediates immunosuppression, impairs thyroid function, and does not prevent renal dysfunction or death [37]. In one study dopamine was associated with an increased risk of death [38]. Authors of the recent international guidelines for management of severe sepsis and septic shock recommend that low-dose dopamine not be used for renal protection [9]. At high doses, dopamine may precipitate supraventricular arrhythmias. The role of non-catecholamine drugs, such as vasopressin, levosimendan, methylene blue, and the phosphodiesterase inhibitors, to support the circulation in sepsis remains to be clarified [17].

The problem of adrenal insufficiency in severe sepsis has focused much interest. Complete adrenal failure is rare in sepsis, but relative adrenal insufficiency is more common. An inadequate response to synthetic corticotrophin (defined as ≤9 μg/dl increase in cortisol level 1 hour after administration of 250 μg ACTH) was found in the majority of patients with septic shock [39]. A 5- to 7-day course of physiologic hydrocortisone doses with subsequent tapering increased the survival rate and shock reversal in patients with vasopressor-dependent septic shock, while short courses of high-dose glucocorticoids decreased patient survival [38]. Two meta-analyses concluded that low dose hydrocortisone for 5 to 11 days in patients with severe sepsis or septic shock significantly reduces the duration of shock and in-hospital mortality [40,41]. One expert opinion suggested that an ACTH stimulation test should be performed and corticosteroid should be started treatment as soon as possible in patients with vasopressor-dependent shock, respiratory failure, and an additional organ failure; subsequently corticosteroids can be discontinued in patients having an adequate response to ACTH [17]. There is disagreement, however, regarding the utility of corticotherapy in patients with sepsis and septic shock and also relative to the use of the ACTH stimulation test to indicate who should receive hydrocortisone treatment. First, adrenal function in the critically ill is a dynamic process, and an appropriate initial adrenal response does not preclude later development of relative adrenal insufficiency [42]. Second, in a number of studies supplementation of corticosteroids did not improve survival in critical illness [43,44]. Authors of the recent international guidelines for management of severe sepsis and septic shock suggested that the ACTH stimulation test not be used to identify the subset of adults with septic shock who should receive hydrocortisone [18].

Nutrition requirements during severe sepsis are also subject to controversies. In general, early enteral nutrition is recommended [17]. Nutritional supplements, such as l-arginine and omega-3 fatty acids, unexpectedly increased the mortality in patients with severe sepsis [45,46]. Furthermore, the indication for strict glucose control in septic patients is controversial. Controlled trials of aggressive glycemic control have provided insufficient evidence to justify subjecting patients to the real risks of iatrogenic hypoglycemia [47]. A meta-analysis of the benefits and risks of tight glucose control in critically ill adults showed that tight glucose control is not associated with significantly reduced hospital mortality but is connected with an increased risk of hypoglycemia [48]. A cautious approach to the treatment of hyperglycemia in patients with sepsis has been recommended, with target blood glucose of 144-162 mg/Dl [47].

Immune dysregulation in sepsis is accompanied by a more pronounced procoagulant state [13]. Patients with severe sepsis should receive deep vein thrombosis prophylaxis unless there are contraindications such as active bleeding, recent intracerebral hemorrhage, thrombocytopenia or severe coagulopathy. Either low-dose unfractionated heparin administered twice or three times per day is recommended or daily low-molecular weight heparin. Unfractionated heparin is preferred over low-molecular weight heparin in patients with moderate to severe renal dysfunction [18]. Also, stress ulcer prophylaxis should be provided using a H2 blocker or proton pump inhibitor [18].

Guidelines

The 2004 guidelines on treatment of sepsis and septic shock have been recently updated [18]. Recommendations were graded according to the quality of evidence from high (A) to very low (D) and according to the strength of recommendations. A strong recommendation (1) indicates that an intervention's desirable effects clearly outweigh its undesirable effects (risk, burden, cost). Weak recommendations (2) indicate that the balance between desirable and undesirable effects is less clear. The grade of strong or weak is considered of greater clinical importance than a difference in letter level of quality of evidence. Key recommendations of the 2008 guidelines include: early goal-directed resuscitation of the septic patient during the first 6 hours after recognition (1C); blood cultures taken before antibiotic therapy (1C); imaging studies performed promptly to confirm potential source of infection (1C); administration of broad-spectrum antibiotic therapy within 1 hour of diagnosis of septic shock (1B) and severe sepsis without septic shock (1D); reassessment of antibiotic therapy with microbiology and clinical data to narrow coverage, when appropriate (1C); an usual 7-10 days of antibiotic therapy guided by clinical response (1D); source control with attention to the balance of risks and benefits of the chosen method (1C); administration of either crystalloid or colloid fluid resuscitation (1B); fluid challenge to restore mean circulating filling pressure (1C); reduction in rate of fluid administration with rising filing pressures (1D); vasopressor preference for norepinephrine or dopamine to maintain an initial target of mean arterial pressure 65 mm Hg or more (1C); dobutamine inotropic therapy when cardiac output remains low despite fluid resuscitation and combined inotropic/vasopressor therapy (1C); stress-dose steroid therapy given only in septic shock after blood pressure is identified to be poorly responsive to fluid and vasopressor therapy (2C); recombinant activated protein C in patients with severe sepsis and high risk for death by clinical assessment (2B except 2C for postoperative patients). In the absence of tissue hypoperfusion, coronary artery disease, or acute hemorrhage, the target hemoglobin should be 7-9 g/dL (1B); a low tidal volume (1B) and limitation of inspiratory plateau pressure strategy (1C) for acute lung injury (ALI)/acute respiratory distress syndrome (ARDS); application of at least a minimal amount of positive end-expiratory pressure in acute lung injury (1C); head of bed elevation in mechanically ventilated patients unless contraindicated (1B); avoiding routine use of pulmonary artery catheters (1A); institution of glycemic control (1B), targeting a blood glucose lower than 150 mg/dL after initial stabilization (2C); equivalency of continuous veno-veno hemofiltration or intermittent hemodialysis (2B); prophylaxis for deep vein thrombosis (1A); use of stress ulcer prophylaxis to prevent upper gastrointestinal bleeding using H2 blockers (1A) or proton pump inhibitors (1B).

Some of the above recommendations may be less suitable for old patients, in particular for frail subjects.

III. EMPIRICAL ANTIBIOTIC TREATMENT OF SEPSIS IN ACUTE GERIATRIC CARE

In our institution, piperacillin-tazobactam is at present the first choice empirical treatment for sepsis of suspected genitourinary origin, for hospital acquired pneumonia, and for sepsis of unknown source. However, if pseudomonas infection is thought to be unlikely, other empiric treatments are considered, for example ertapenem. The efficiency of this routine is illustrated by the case histories of three patients who developed sepsis, while hospitalized for different causes in the geriatric ward during the first week of August 2008. There may be an extra benefit of this routine. Reports in the literature suggest that empiric treatment of sepsis with piperacillin-tazobactam might be a suitable strategy to decrease endemic CEP resistance (controlled gene expression following ectopic integration into the chromosome) by K. pneumoniae and P. mirabilis [49].

Case 1 - Piperacillin-Tazobactam for Suspected Hospital Acquired Pneumonia

An 82-year-old woman with Streptococcus viridans endocarditis, severe aortic stenosis, and left heart failure was improving after 2 weeks of intravenous penicillin treatment, when she became confused, with 39.3°C fever and dyspnea. Pulmonary congestion and bilateral alveolar infiltrates were noted on chest X rays. Blood and urine cultures were obtained. In suspecting hospital acquired pneumonia, empirical treatment with piperacillin-tazobactam was started and furosemide was administered intravenously. The fever subsided within 36 hours, the delirium and dyspnea remitted, and the alveolar infiltrates disappeared on chest X rays. E. coli was retrieved from the urine culture, more than 100.000 colonies/cc, resistant to piperacillin-tazobactam but sensitive to ertapenem. The fast clearance of bilateral pulmonary infiltrates after administration of furosemide demonstrated that heart failure was their cause. The diagnosis of hospital-acquired pneumonia turned out to be wrong and urosepsis was the final diagnosis. Though sepsis was obviously remitting, piperacillin-tazobactam was exchanged to ertapenem, which was administered for 5 days. Thereafter, a 4 week course of penicillin treatment for endocarditis was completed. She was discharged in good condition. Piperacillin-tazobactam was efficient as first line treatment of sepsis in vivo, though bacteriology laboratory data showed a different sensitivity in vitro.

Case 2 - Piperacillin-Tazobactam Efficient in Culture-Negative Sepsis

A 91-year-old woman was in good general health until recently, when she was hospitalized with myocardial infarction and E. coli urinary tract infection. Two weeks later, ischemic gangrene of the toe developed and MRSA osteomyelitis of the first metatarsal bone was diagnosed. After surgical debridement of the necrotic tissues she was transferred to our geriatric ward for long-term intravenous vancomycin treatment. Three weeks on vancomycin she became unexpectedly obtunded, hypotensive and temperature increased to 39.6°C. In suspecting sepsis, treatment with piperacillin-tazobactam was started. A few hours later she passed two tarry black stools, became anuric, and was transferred to the intensive care unit. Defeverness followed soon, but renal failure developed with decline of the creatinine clearance to 29 ml/min/m^2. Numerous blood and urine cultures were negative, so empirical treatment with piperacillin-tazobactam was continued. The vancomicin dose was adjusted to the diminished renal function. After completion of a 14 day course, piperacillin-tazobactam was discontinued and specimen for blood and urine cultures were obtained. A spike of fever 39.1°C followed. Piperacillin-tazobactam was re-instituted and the temperature returned to normal, along with hemodynamic stability and improvement of mentation. Again, urine and blood cultures did not show any growth. On further evaluation, echocardiography showed no evidence of valvular vegetations and computerized tomography did not reveal an infectious focus. There was no recurrence of sepsis. The patient refused to undergo gastrointestinal endoscopy.

In this patient, piperacillin-tazobactam was an efficient initial treatment of sepsis and again efficient at the time of sepsis recurrence. No pathogen could be recovered on numerous cultures.

Case 3 - Piperacillin-Tazobactam Unexpectedly Effective in Treatment of Septicemia with Carbapenem-Resistant Klebsiella Pneumoniae

An 87-year-old man was admitted to the geriatric ward with delirium. Lately he suffered of diarrhea, and Campylobacter jejuni was recovered from his stool. The diarrhea was successfully treated with ciprofloxacin 500 mg orally b.i.d. for 5 days. The patient's medical history included chronic lymphoid leukemia, arterial hypertension, chronic atrial fibrillation, chronic renal failure and folate deficiency. The latest medications were metoprolol, furosemide, folic acid and ferrous sulphate. At the time of admission to our ward the temperature was 36.5°C, heart rate 74 bpm, respiratory rate 18 breaths per minute, supine BP 160/94 mm Hg, and oxygen saturation 92% on ambient air. He had an altered level of consciousness and disorganized thinking, fluctuating during the course of the day. The body temperature was normal. Routine laboratory tests showed normocytic anemia and moderate renal failure (hematocrit 34%, blood urea nitrogen 45 mg/dL, serum creatinine 1.6 mg/dL). Range-of-motion exercises, assisted ambulation and low-impact resistive exercises of lower extremities were started; the regular medications were continued. On the second week after admission the occurrence of a vesicular eruption characteristic of trigeminal zona zoster was noticed on the patient's face. The temperature remained normal. He was treated with intravenous acyclovir and made an uneventful recovery. The third week in the ward the patient became sleepy, had shaking chills and the temperature rose to 39.4°C. There was neither cough, diarrhea, urinary frequency or skin eruption. The white blood cell count increased to 16.000/mm^3 with 68% neutrophils, the C reactive protein increased to 84 mg/L; urinalysis and chest X rays were unrewarding. Blood and urine cultures were obtained and empiric treatment with piperacillin-tazobactam was started. The spiking fever remitted on the third day of antibiotic treatment. Urinalysis and urine cultures were unremarkable. Two of the three blood cultures grew carbapenem-resistant Klebsiella pneumoniae, which was insensitive in vitro to piperacillin-tazobactam. The antibiotic susceptibilities of the isolate were confirmed at another laboratory. Because definitive recognition of carbapenem resistance in Klebsiella pneumoniae can be ascertained only by molecular methods [50,51], the isolate was subjected to randomly amplified polymorphic DNA (RAPD) polymerase chain reaction (PCR), PCR amplification and sequencing of the KPC genes. The PCR and sequencing of the KPC genes endorsed the bacteriologic diagnosis by identifying the blaKPC gene in the specimen.

Once more piperacillin-tazobactam was efficient as empirical first line treatment of sepsis, but, as it turned out, it was effective against carbapenem-resistant Klebsiella pneumoniae. The bacteriologic diagnosis was verified by PCR technique, with sensitivity and specificity of the assay approaching 100% [52]. When results of microbiology become available, antibiotic therapy treatment was changed to tigecycline and the patient made an uneventful recovery. The clinical remission on piperacillin-tazobactam was impressive and surprising, a posteriori. That carbapenem-resistant Klebsiella pneumoniae responded well to piperacillin-tazobactam treatment in vivo is not clearly understood.

Learning points:

- The choice of empiric antimicrobial therapy of sepsis depends on the clinical syndrome, underlying disease, susceptibility patterns of pathogens that previously have been documented to colonize or infect the patient, and drug intolerances.
- An emerging consensus emphasizes the importance of local unit-specific antimicrobial sensitivity data in selection of empiric antibiotic treatment.
- It is generally recommended that de-escalation to the most appropriate single therapy should be performed as soon as the susceptibility profile is known.

IV. Vancomycin Treatment for MRSA Infections

In 1958, vancomycin was introduced in clinical practice as an agent active against penicillin-resistant Staphylococcus aureus. A few years later, when the new penicillinase-resistant β-lactams methicillin and cephalothin became available, the use of vancomycin decreased, mainly because of and the high rate of toxicity of the initial vancomycin preparations. Later manufacturing procedures improved vancomycin purity and from this time a conmtinual rise in vancomycin use has occurred [53]. New agents with broad Gram positive activity have emerged but none is evidently superior to vancomicin.

Vancomycin is most often prescribed for treatment of serious infections caused by β-lactam–resistant Gram positive organisms, infections caused by Gram positive organisms in patients with serious allergy to β-lactams, and antibiotic-associated colitis that has not responded to metronidazole or that is severe and potentially life threatening. The bactericidal activity of vancomycin is concentration independent once a concentration of four or five times the MIC for the organism is reached. Vancomycin concentrations achieved in serum in normal volunteers 2 hours after an intravenous dose of 1g are around 25 µg/mL; these levels decrease to 2 µg/mL by 12 hours. Vancomycin is primarily excreted unchanged via the kidneys by glomerular filtration. A linear correlation between creatinine clearance and vancomycin levels is recognized. Vancomycin half life in adults with normal renal function is 4–11 hours, but increases to 6-10 days in advanced reanl failure [54].

Vancomycin treatment is usually started with a fixed loading dose of 25 mg/kg body weight followed by a maintenance dose that typically is 1g at 12 hour intervals in an adult with normal renal function. In patients with decreased creatinine clearance, nomograms and formulas are used to determine the dosing schedule. A convenient approach is to lengthen the interval between two consecutive 1g doses of vancomycin, according to the equation: Interval = normal interval x (86 mL/min ÷ [0.689 × creatinine clearance mL/min + 3.66]). This treatment regimen should result in an approximate vancomycin serum peak value 30 µg/mL and a trough value 7.5 µg/mL. A meta-analysis of randomised controlled trials comparing intermittent intravenous administration with continuous intravenous infusion of the same total dose of vancomycin showed that continuous intravenous infusion may be more efficient [55]. The recommendation to monitor vancomycin serum concentration to optimize efficiency with minimal toxicity is the subject of debate [56-58].

Case 4– Vancomycin Nephrotoxicity

Monitoring vancomycin serum concentration is not always helpful in preventing vancomycin toxicity. This is illustrated in the patient presented in detail in the chapter 'Normotensive shock'. Succinctly, a 72-year-old man presenting with MRSA septicemia and L1-L2 discitis was admitted for long-term antibiotic treatment. The patient's medical history included arterial hypertension, ischemic heart disease, congestive heart failure, diabetes mellitus, and mild renal failure. On physical examination, the patient was cachectic, the blood pressure 182/84 mmHg, the heart rate 76 bpm, respirations 16 per minute. maximum temperature 37.6°C, and oxygen saturation 92% on room air. There was hepatojugualar reflux and grade 1 ankle edema. Laboratory tests were remarkable for C reactive protein 230 mg/L, serum creatinine 1.6 mg/dl, albumin 2.8 g/l. The estimated creatinine clearance according to the Modification of Diet in Renal Disease equation and Cockcroft-Gault equation was 45 mL/min/1.73 m^2 and 30 mL/min/1.73 m^2, respectively. Treatment with intravenous vancomycin 1g at 24 hour intervals was administered. Vancomycin trough levels were measured twice per week and were found satisfactory, between 5 and 8 µg/mL. The patient continued to receive his current medications, including aspirin 100 mg/day, carvedilol 12.5 mg/day, ramipril 5 mg/day, furosemide 40 mg/day, spironolacton 12.5 mg/day, simvastatin 20 mg/day and insulin.

Thirty days on vancomycin treatment, the temperature was normal and the C reactive protein decreased to 18 mg/L. However, the patient's heart failure deteriorated, with generalized edema and pulmonary congestion. The estimated creatinine clearance was unchanged. Furosemide i.v drip 160 mg/24 hours was administered. Six days later the serum creatinine had risen to 3 mg/dl and the BUN to 110 mg/dl. The urinary sediment was unremarkable. There was no change in the blood pressure, varying between 124-160/70-82 mmHg. On diagnosing the severe deterioration in renal function, treatment with vancomycin, furosemid and ramipril was discontinued, and rifampicin treatment was instituted. Gradually, over a period of 10 days the creatinine decreased to 2.6 mg/dl and the BUN to 32 mg/dl. In this patient, advanced age, poor nutritional state, hypoalbuminemia, chronic renal failure, and use of a loop diuretic were preexisting risk factors of vancomycin nephrotoxicity. When additional risk factors came in action, specifically exacerbation of heart failure and administration of large doses of furosemide, an acute worsening of renal failure occurred. Monitoring the serum vancomycin concentration twice weekly was insufficient to predict nephrotoxicity.

Nephrotoxicity associated with vancomycin has been reported since the beginning of its clinical use, and thought to be related, at least in part, to impurities in the early preparations [59]. Modern prospectively designed studies reported an incidence of renal functional impairment between zero and 7%. However, when vancomycin was co-administered with an aminoglycoside the nephrotoxicity rate increased to 14-20% [60,61]. Acute interstitial nephritis associated with vancomycin use has also been reported [62]. Several studies have shoed a higher rate of nephrotoxicity in subjects with vancomycin trough levels greater than 10 µg/mL or 15 µg/mL and investigators proposed that measurement of vancomycin levels in serum should be used to optimize therapy [63]. Others have not found a close correlation between vancomycin serum levels and nephrotoxicity [64,65], as opposed to the fair prediction of toxicity by aminoglycosides serum levels.

An approach to minimize the monitoring of vancomycin serum levels was evaluated in a prospective work comparing two treatment modalities. In the first group, patients with the minimized monitoring regimen were dosed by a nomogram and had the regimens adjusted based on actual body weight, estimated creatinine clearance, and a targeted trough concentration of 5-20 microg/ml; a single trough serum concentration was drawn only after 5 or more days of therapy. In the second group, vancomycin levels were frequently tested and serum peak and trough concentrations served to adjust the daily dose of the antibiotic. No differences were found between the two groups with respect to improvement and cure rates, days to eradication, and nephrotoxicity. Considerable cost savings were achieved for patients dosed by nomogram compared with patients dosed by pharmacokinetics [64]. Based on this data, a number of investigators have taken position against the routine measurement of vancomycin serum levels [65].

There are special circumstances when it is prudent to more frequently measure vancomycin concentrations (Table 1), including patients concomitantly receiving another nephrotoxic agent especially aminoglycosides; patients receiving high-dose vancomycin; subjects undergoing hemodialysis; patients with morbid obesity; in the face of rapidly changing or unpredictable renal function; during prolonged vancomycin therapy (longer than 10 days); concurrent or sequential use of systemic or topical potentially nephrotoxic drugs - cisplatin, cephaloridine, gentamicin, kanamycin, amikacin, neomycin, polymixin B, colistin, paromomycin, streptomycin, tobramycin and viomycin [66,67]. Nephrotoxicity is more frequent in elderly patients than in the young; in one study nephrotoxicity of vancomycin vas noticed in 18.9% of the elderly patients versus 7.8% of younger patients [68]. Concurrent loop diuretic use is significantly associated with vancomycin-associated nephrotoxicity (relative risk 5.0)[66]. In patients receiving continuous infusion vancomycin, a serum steady-state vancomycin concentration ≥28 mg/L increases markedly the risk (OR 21)[69]. A significantly increased risk of nephrotoxicity was observed among patients receiving ≥4 g/day vancomycin/day (34.6% nephrotoxicity), compared with those receiving <4 g vancomycin/day (10.9%), and compared to patients receiving linezolid (6.7%) [70].

Under special circumstances when serum vancomycin will be measured, patients should have received a minimum of three vancomycin doses or 48 hours of therapy before testing. Samples for trough concentrations should be obtained within 30 minutes of the next scheduled dose. Samples for peak concentrations should be obtained one hour after the end of the infusion. Traditional trough concentrations of 5 to 10 microgram/mL [71,72] are being reconsidered in view of increasing minimum inhibitory concentrations of staphylococci to vancomycin. Trough concentrations of 10 to 15 microgram/mL are generally recommended [55], but for treatment of deep-seated staphylococcal infections such as endocarditis, prosthetic joint infections, CNS infections trough 15 to 20 microgram/mL are recommended [64,73].

Learning points:

- Most important among risk factors of vancomycin nephrotoxicity are prolonged treatment, concomitant administration of other nephrotoxic agents, advanced patient age, low serum albumin, poor nutritional status, dehydration, kidney disease, shock, and administration of loop diuretics.
- Minimal monitoring of vancomycin therapy by taking a single trough serum concentration after 5 or more days of therapy is safe, as long as the patient is hemodynamically stable.
- In patients with rapidly changing renal function, day-to-day monitoring of serum levels may be advisable. Table 1. Risk factors of vancomycin nephrotoxicity

Advanced patient age
Poor nutritional status
Decreased serum albumin
Dehydration
Hypercalcemia
Kidney disease
Shock
Prolonged treatment
Steady-state vancomycin concentration ≥28 mg/L
Concomitant administration of other nephrotoxic agents
Leukemia
Rapidly fatal illness
Pneumonia
Pleural effusion
Liver disease
Obesity

Case 5 - Spurious Vancomycin Toxicity

This case has been described in detail elsewhere [74]. A 56-year-old man was admitted for treatment of sternal osteomyelitis subsequent to coronary artery bypass surgery. On vancomycin treatment, the initial trough vancomycin level was 10.3 µg/mL. Later during the course of treatment, the access to superficial veins became difficult and a central PermCath venous catheter was inserted via the axillary vein to provide venous access. A few days later, the trough vancomycin level was 62 µg/mL in a blood sample obtained via the PermCath. The patient was symptom free and the plasma creatinine was 0.8 mg/dL. Vancomycin administration was discontinued. Sixteen hours later, vancomycin trough was 120 µg/mL in blood drawn trough the PermCath. On the same day, repeated sampling produced vancomycin trough level 43.4 µg/mL in blood drawn via the PermCath, while blood drawn at the same time by puncturing the femoral vein showed vancomycin 10.1 µg/mL. This observation was replicated on the following day. Flushing the PermCath with 10 ml or 50 ml of saline did not eliminate the vancomycine from the line. Thus, samples of saline removed from the line (after its rinsing out) or blood removed via the line contained high concentrations of vancomycin. Unvariably, 'toxic' vancomycine levels were related solely to the PermCath line. The simple and obvious explanation to spuriously toxic vancomycin levels in this patient may be that vancomycin was adhering to the venous catheter.

Learning point:

- Spuriously 'toxic' vancomycin levels may arise by drawing blood through venous lines.

Case 6 – Vancomycin Induced Neutropenia

A 79-year-old woman received vancomycin after removal of an infected hip prosthesis. MRSA was cultured in a specimen acquired from the wound at the time of surgery. The patient's medical history included osteoarthritis and arterial hypertension. Her regular medications were ramipril, hydrochlorothiazide, simvastatin, aspirin and oxycodone. Vancomycin treatment was administered intravenously 1g at 36 hour intervals and the once measured trough level was 2.2µg/mL. The serum creatinine was 1.2 mg/Dl. The clinical response was favorable; after 4 weeks of treatment the temperature was normal and the C reactive protein was 12 mg/L. At this time point, a fall in the white blood cell count was witnessed from 11200/mm^3 with 82% neutrophils to 3400/mm^3 white blood cell with 1150/mm^3 neutrophils and no band forms. The hemoglobin was 11g/dL and the platelets 230000/mm^3, essentially unchanged. The C reactive protein was 10.2 mg/L. Common causes of selective neutropenia could be eliminated, mainly infections and a variety of drugs, thus the possibility that vancomycin caused this patient's neutopenia was considered. Vancomycin was replaced with rifampin and fusidic acid. Within 3 days the neutrophil count increased to 1620/mm3 and after one week to 3100/mm^3, the total white blood cells were 6040/mm^3. The subsequent course was uneventful.

Although unusual, neutropenia associated with vancomycin therapy may occur, with a frequency of about 1% to 2%. This rate increases with long-term vancomycin administration. Neutropenia usually resolves after discontinuation of the drug. In the case described by Mackett et al. [75] neutropenia was noticed on day 17 of vancomycin treatment, it progressed over the next 3 days, and after discontinuation of vancomycin a rise in the neutrophil count occurred within 5 days of discontinuation. This is not unlike to the course of neutropenia in the patient treated by us. In a patient described by Koo et al. [76], severe leukopenia developed on vancomycin with the presence of only occasional neutrophils in the peripheral blood. On discontinuation of vancomycin, the leukocyte and neutrophil counts promptly increased with full recovery after a week. Subsequently, the patient was restarted on a five-day course of vancomycin at a lower dose, that was uneventful, without recurrence of neutropenia. The latter observation is in disagreement with the commonly held concept that an immunologic mechanism may be responsible for the reaction. Vancomycin-induced neutropenia may occur more often than previously reported. The rate was 13% in patients treated with vancomycin for a mean of 6.2 months [77]. In another study, 14 of 114 (12%) patients treated with vancomycin developed vancomycin-induced neutropenia, including 4 cases with absolute neutrophil counts ≤500 cells/mm^3. The mean duration of vancomycin therapy and time to neutropenia were 32 days. Resolution of vancomycin-induced neutropenia occurred promptly after discontinuation. There was no correlation between total vancomycin doses and serum concentrations with development of neutropenia. The authors concluded that clinicians should monitor the blood cell count at least weekly in patients receiving vancomycin therapy for longer than 2 weeks [78]. Vancomycin-induced neutropenia was reversible by administration of granulocyte colony-stimulating factor in two patients receiving long-term vancomycin therapy as outpatients [79].

Learning points:

- Neutropenia may occur on long-term vancomycin treatment.
- Vancomycin-induced neutropenia may be severe.
- Resolution occurs promptly after discontinuation of vancomycin.
- Blood cell count should be monitored at least weekly in patients receiving vancomycin therapy for longer than 2 weeks.

The recognition of the shortcomings of vancomycin as an antistaphylococcal agent, together with the availability of alternative effective antistaphylococcal antibiotics, has led to a reassessment of its role therapeutics. Evidence suggests that vancomycin may be inferior to some comparator agents in the treatment of infections due to MRSA. This, together with the problem of heteroresistance to vancomycin, as well as poor tissue penetration after its systemic administration, presents potential obstacles to the successful therapy of S. aureus infections with vancomycin. While it was implied that these problems may be overcome by administration of much higher doses of vancomycin, the efficacy and safety of the proposed high dosre schedule remains to be proven by randomized clinical trials.

In the last few years new anti-MRSA drugs have been registered [80,81], such are linezolid the most widely used new anti-MRSA agent, quinupristin-dalfopristin, daptomycin, a novel lipopeptide, active on germs both in the replicating and in the resting phase, and tigecycline, the first approved glycylcycline. Other drugs from different classes are in development and will further enhance in the next few years our therapeutic armamentarium: three glycopeptides (dalbavancin, telavancin, and oritavancin), two broad spectrum cephalosporins, ceftobiprole and ceftaroline, iclaprim, a diaminopyrimidine, as well as a carbapenem, CS-023/RO-4908463, and adjuvant therapies such as the monoclonal antibody tefibazumab. Despite the fact that these newer agents have been compared with vancomycin in trials only designed to demonstrate noninferiority, some potential evidence of superiority over vancomycin has emerged.

V. CONTAINMENT OF INFECTION WITH RESISTANT STRAINS

Antimicrobial resistance in health care-associated pathogens is a growing problem [22,26,82]. A recent shift in the epidemiological profile of methicillin-resistant Staphylococcus aureus has resulted in increased rates of health care-associated infections and also in community-associated infections [83]. There is growing resistance of Staphylococcus aureus to vancomycin [84]. The rate of vancomycin resistance among Enterococcus faecium has also increased [85]. Multidrug resistance in Pseudomonas aeruginosa is rising. Carbapenem-resistant Klebsiella strains have emerged [22]. Acinetobacter species are increasingly resistant to carbapenems and third-generation cephalosporins. A hypervirulent strain of Clostridium difficile has increased resistance to fluoroquinolones. An alarming escalation of hospital-acquired infections due to multi-drug resistant Gram negative bacteria has occurred. Pseudomonas aeruginosa or Acinetobacter baumanii isolates found to be resistant to all commonly used antibiotics are now treated with older drugs such as colistin or combinations of antibiotics.

In acute geriatric care, skillful use of antibiotics and the undertaking of infection containing are difficult, perhaps more than in other settings. Principles of containment of infection with resistant bacterial strains have been summarized under the auspices of the Centers for Disease Control and Prevention's in 2006 [86]. In essence, persistence of the resistant strain in a healthcare setting is dependent on the presence of vulnerable patients, antimicrobial use, increased potential for transmission from colonized or infected patients, and implementation of prevention efforts. Patients vulnerable to colonization and infection include those with severe disease, especially those with compromised host defenses from underlying medical conditions, recent surgery, or indwelling medical devices. Multidrug-resistant organisms are carried from one person to another via the hands of health care providers. Hands are easily contaminated during the process of care-giving or from contact with environmental surfaces in close proximity to the patient. Without adherence to hand hygiene and glove use, health care providers are likely to transmit multidrug-resistant organisms to patients. Universal precautions should be used for all patients during contact with blood, body fluids, or secretions, i.e. wearing gloves, spectacles and impermeable gowns if aerosol or splash is likely. Aggressive isolation is recommended to restrict spread of resistant organisms and their plasmids for MRSA, VREF and highly resistant gram-negative organisms. The contact precautions can be discontinued when three or more surveillance cultures for the target multi-drug resistant organism are repeatedly negative over the course of a week or two in a patient who has not received antimicrobial therapy for several weeks [86]. Thus, strategies to increase and monitor adherence are important components of multidrug-resistant organisms control programs [86].

For containment of infection with resistant strains, application of barrier precautions has been shown to be highly efficient [87-89]. Here are some examples. A control program to prevent the spread of multi-resistant bacteria in a teaching hospital focused on methicillin-resistant MRSA and enterobacteriaceae producing extended-spectrum beta-lactamases (ESBL); the intervention was based on washing hands with antiseptic soaps, wearing disposable gloves and gowns, and identifying carriers of multi-resistant bacteria [89]. The incidence of infection decreased by 17.9% for MRSA and by 54.9% for ESBL. The decrease of the incidence concerned both resistant and susceptible strains. In nursing homes, aggressive containment practices are also efficient in reducing colonization rates. In a nursing home, the initial colonization rate with MRSA was 52% among residents. To decrease colonization and infection rates and to prevent the introduction of additional colonized patients into the closed environment, a program was initiated comprising total population and staff surveillance and aggressive containment measures (contact isolation, baths with chlorhexagluconate, treatment of nasal carriers with bacitracin and treatment of both colonized and infected patients). This was followed by maintenance measures of screening new admissions for MRSA with contact isolation and treatment for positive cases as described during the aggressive phase. Total population surveillance was repeated after one year. After one year the colonization rate dropped to 2% and the infection rate to 1.4%, no employees were colonized with MRSA. This reduction was maintained over time [90].

Elaboration of institutional guidelines for prevention of transmission of multidrug-resistant organisms are an imperative need. Examples of such guidelines [91] recommend performance of active surveillance cultures for patients after admission to health care facilities or to high-risk-patient care units, to detect colonization with target multidrug-resistant organisms. Patients who are colonized with these potential pathogens are placed under contact precautions to prevent transmission to other patients. Such screening programs raise ethical considerations of restricted autonomy, and require education of patients, family members and visitors. Yet, there is a lack of consensus among recommended infection control guidelines [92] and little is known about the occurrence of multidrug-resistant organisms among home care and hospice patients [8].

Application of the guidelines for management of multidrug-resistant organisms may be particularly difficult in the setting of acute geriatric ward, where patients are often confused or demented, and their elderly visitors may have limitations in understanding the recommendations and in cooperation. It is a difficult to achieve must.

REFERENCES

[1]   American College of Chest Physicians/Society of Critical Care Medicine Consensus Conference Committee : Definitions for sepsis and organ failure and guidelines for the use of innovative therapies in sepsis. Crit. Care Med., 1992, 20, 864-874.

[2]   Martin, GS; Mannino, DM; Eaton, S; et al: The epidemiology of sepsis in the United States from 1979 through 2000. N. Engl. J. Med., 2003, 348, 1546-1554.

[3]   O'Brien JM, Jr; Ali, NA; Aberegg, SK; Abraham, E. Sepsis. Am. J. Med., 2007, 120, 1012-1022.

[4]   Shapiro, NI; Howell, MD; Talmor, D; Lahey, D; Ngo, L; Buras, J; Wolfe, RE; Weiss, JW; Lisbon, A. Implementation and outcomes of the Multiple Urgent Sepsis Therapies (MUST) protocol. Crit. Care Med., 2006, 34, 1025-1032.

[5]   Kortgen, A; Niederprum, P; Bauer, M. Implementation of an evidence-based "standard operating procedure" and outcome in septic shock. Crit. Care Med., 2006, 34, 943-949.

[6]   Martin, GS; Mannino, DM; Moss, M. The effect of age on the development and outcome of adult sepsis. Crit. Care Med., 2006, 34, 15-21.

[7]   Siegel, RE. Emerging gram-negative antibiotic resistance: daunting challenges, declining sensitivities, and dire consequences. Respir. Care., 2008, 53, 471-479.

[8]   McGoldrick, M; Rhinehart, E. Managing multidrug-resistant organisms in home care and hospice: surveillance, prevention, and control. *Home Healthc Nurse.*, 2007, 25, 580-586.

[9]   Rittirsch, D; Flierl, MA; Ward, PA. Harmful molecular mechanisms in sepsis. *Nat. Rev. Immunol.*, 2008, 8, 776-787.

[10] Lyn-Kew, K; Standiford, TJ. Immunosuppression in sepsis. *Curr. Pharm. Des.* 2008, 14, 1870-1881.

[11] Wang, L; Bastarache, JA; Ware, LB. The coagulation cascade in sepsis. *Curr. Pharm. Des.*, 2008,14, 1860-1869.

[12] Crouser, E; Exline, M; Knoell, D; Wewers, MD. Sepsis: links between pathogen sensing and organ damage. *Curr. Pharm. Des.*, 2008, 14, 1840-1852.

[13] Opal, SM; Girard, TD; Ely, EW. The immunopathogenesis of sepsis in elderly patients. *Clin. Infect. Dis.*, 2005, 41 Suppl 7, S504-512.

[14] Lever, A; Mackenzie, I. Sepsis: definition, epidemiology, and diagnosis. *BMJ.*, 2007, 335, 879-883

[15] Lee, CC; Chen, SY; Chang, IJ; Chen, SC; Wu, SC. Comparison of clinical manifestations and outcome of community-acquired bloodstream infections among the oldest old, elderly, and adult patients. *Medicine.* (Baltimore) 2007, 86, 138-144.

[16] Payeras, A; García-Gasalla, M; Garau, M; Juan, I; Roca, M; Pareja, A; Cifuentes, C; Homar, F; Gallegos, C; Bassa, A. Bacteremia in very elderly patients: risk factors, clinical characteristics and mortality. *Enferm. Infecc. Microbiol. Clin.*, 2007, 25, 612-618.

[17] Mackenzie, I; Lever, A. Management of sepsis. *BMJ*, 2007, 335, 929-932. Englehart, MS; Schreiber, MA. Measurement of acid-base resuscitation endpoints: lactate, base deficit, bicarbonate or what? *Curr. Opin. Crit. Care.*, 2006, 12, 569-574.

[18] Dellinger, RP; Levy, MM; Carlet, JM; Bion, J; Parker, MM; Jaeschke, R; Reinhart, K; Angus, DC; Brun-Buisson, C; Beale, R; Calandra, T; Dhainaut, JF; Gerlach, H; Harvey, M; Marini, JJ; Marshall, J; Ranieri, M; Ramsay, G; Sevransky, J; Thompson, BT; Townsend, S; Vender, JS; Zimmerman, JL; Vincent, JL. Surviving Sepsis Campaign: international guidelines for management of severe sepsis and septic shock: 2008. *Crit. Care Med.*, 2008, 36, 296-327.

[19] Murray, PR; ed-in-chief, Manual of Clinical Microbiology, 8th ed.. Washington, DC, ASM Press, 2003.

[20] Leibovici, L; Shraga, I; Drucker, M; et al: The benefit of appropriate empirical antibiotic treatment in patients with bloodstream infection. *J. Intern. Med.*, 1998, 244, 379–386.

[21] Ibrahim, EH; Sherman, G; Ward, S; et al: The influence of inadequate antimicrobial treatment of bloodstream infections on patient outcomes in the ICU setting. *Chest.*, 2000, 118, 146–155.

[22] Nicasio, AM; Kuti, JL; Nicolau, DP. The current state of multidrug-resistant gram-negative bacilli in North America. *Pharmacotherapy.*, 2008, 28, 235-249.

[23] Cunha, BA. Sepsis and septic shock: selection of empiric antimicrobial therapy. *Critical Care Clinics.*, 2008, 24, 313-334.

[24] Cosgrove, SE; Carmeli, Y. The impact of antimicrobial resistance on health and economic outcomes. *Clin. Infect. Dis.*, 2003, 36, 1433–1437.

[25] Kaul, DR; Collins, CD; Hyzy, RC. New developments in antimicrobial use in sepsis. *Curr. Pharm. Des.*, 2008, 14, 1912-1920.

[26] Blot, S; Depuydt, P; Vandewoude, K; De Bacquer, D. Measuring the impact of multidrug resistance in nosocomial infection. *Curr. Opin. Infect. Dis.*, 2007, 20, 391-396.

[27] Lee, SC; Huang, SS; Lee, CW; Fung, CP; Lee, N; Shieh, WB; Siu, LK. Comparative antimicrobial susceptibility of aerobic and facultative bacteria from community-acquired bacteremia to ertapenem in Taiwan. *BMC Infect. Dis.*, 2007, 17, 79.

[28] Fan, E; Stewart, TE. Albumin in critical care: SAFE, but worth its salt? *Crit. Care.*, 2004, 8, 297-299.

[29] Liberati, A; Moja, L; Moschetti, I; Gensini, GF; Gusinu, R. Human albumin solution for resuscitation and volume expansion in critically ill patients. *Intern. Emerg. Med.*, *2006*, 1, 243-245.

[30] Lima, A; Bakker, J. Noninvasive monitoring of peripheral perfusion. *Intensive Care Med.*, 2005, 31, 1316-26.

[31] Englehart, MS; Schreiber, MA. Measurement of acid-base resuscitation endpoints: lactate, base deficit, bicarbonate or what? *Curr. Opin. Crit. Care.*, 2006, 12, 569-574.

[32] Ypenburg, C; Bax, JJ; van der Wall, EE; Schalij, MJ; van Erven, L. Intrathoracic impedance monitoring to predict decompensated heart failure. *Am. J. Cardiol.*, 2007, 99, 554-557.

[33] Adamicza, A; Tutsek, L; Nagy, S. Changes in transthoracic electrical impedance during endotoxemia in dogs. *Acta Physiol. Hung.*, 1997-1998, 85, 291-302.

[34] Chytra, I; Pradl, R; Bosman, R; Pelnár, P; Kasal, E; Zidková, A. Esophageal Doppler-guided fluid management decreases blood lactate levels in multiple-trauma patients: a randomized controlled trial. *Crit. Care.*, 2007, 11, R24.

[35] Uchino, S; Bellomo, R; Morimatsu, H; Sugihara, M; French, C; Stephens, D; Wendon, J; Honore, P; Mulder, J; Turner, A; the PAC/PiCCO Use and Likelihood of Success Evaluation [PULSE] Study Group. Pulmonary artery catheter versus pulse contour analysis: a prospective epidemiological study. *Crit. Care.*, 2006, 10, R174.

[36] Elkayam, U; Tien MH, Ng; Hatamizadeh, P; Janmohamed, M; Mehra, A. Renal vasodilatory action of dopamine in patients with heart failure Magnitude of effect and site of action. *Circulation.*, 2008, 117, 200-205.

[37] Friedrich, JO; Adhikari, N; Herridge, MS; Beyene, J. Meta-Analysis: Low-Dose Dopamine Increases Urine Output but Does Not Prevent Renal Dysfunction or Death. *Ann. Intern. Med.*, 2005, 142, 510-524.

[38] Sakr, Y; Reinhart, K; Vincent, JL; Sprung, CL; Moreno, R; Ranieri, VM; De Backer, D; Payen, D. Does dopamine administration in shock influence outcome? Results of the Sepsis Occurrence in Acutely Ill Patients (SOAP) Study. *Crit. Care Med.*, 2006, 34, 589-597.

[39] de Jong, MF; Beishuizen, A; Spijkstra, JJ; Groeneveld, AB. Relative adrenal insufficiency as a predictor of disease severity, mortality, and beneficial effects of corticosteroid treatment in septic shock. *Crit. Care Med.*, 2007, 35, 1896-903.

[40] Minneci, PC; Deans, KJ; Banks, SM; Eichacker, PQ; Natanson, C. Meta-analysis: the effect of steroids on survival and shock during sepsis depends on the dose. *Ann. Intern. Med.*, 2004, 141, 47-56.

[41] Burry, LD; Wax, RS. Role of corticosteroids in septic shock. *Ann. Pharmacother.*, 2004, 38, 464-472.

[42] Guzman, JA; Guzman, CB. Adrenal exhaustion in septic patients with vasopressor dependency. *J. Crit. Care.*, 2007, 22, 319-323.

[43] Rady, MY; Johnson, DJ; Patel, B; Larson, J; Helmers, R. Cortisol levels and corticosteroid administration fail to predict mortality in critical illness: the confounding effects of organ dysfunction and sex. *Arch. Surg.*, 2005, 140, 661-668.

[44] Sprung, CL; Annane, D; Briegel, J. Corticosteroid therapy of septic shock (CORTICUS). Abstr. *Am. Rev. Respir. Crit. Care Med.*, 2007, 175, A507

[45] Beale, RJ; Sherry, T; Lei, K; Campbell-Stephen, L; McCook, J; Smith, J; Venetz, W; Alteheld, B; Stehle, P; Schneider, H. Early enteral supplementation with key pharmaconutrients improves Sequential Organ Failure Assessment score in critically ill patients with sepsis: outcome of a randomized, controlled, double-blind trial. *Crit. Care Med.*, 2006, 34, 2325-2333.

[46] Pontes-Arruda, A; Aragão, AM; Albuquerque, JD. Effects of enteral feeding with eicosapentaenoic acid, gamma-linolenic acid, and antioxidants in mechanically ventilated patients with severe sepsis and septic shock. *Care Med.*, 2008, 36, 131-144.

[47] Henderson, WR; Chittock, DR; Dhingra, VK; Ronco, JJ. Hyperglycemia in acutely ill emergency patients - cause or effect? *CJEM.*, 2006, 8, 339-343.

[48] Wiener, RS; Wiener, DC; Larson, RJ. Benefits and risks of tight glucose control in critically ill adults. *A meta-analysis JAMA.*, 2008, 300, 933-944.

[49] Bantar, C; Vesco, E; Heft, C; Salamone, F; Krayeski, M; Gomez, H; Coassolo, MA; Fiorillo, A; Franco, D; Arango, C; Duret, F; Oliva, ME. Replacement of broad-spectrum cephalosporins by piperacillin-tazobactam: impact on sustained high rates of bacterial resistance. *Antimicrob. Agents Chemother.*, 2004, 48, 392-395.

[50] Babini, GS; Yuan, M; Hall, LM; Livermore, DM. Variable susceptibility to piperacillin/tazobactam amongst Klebsiella spp. with extended-spectrum beta-lactamases. *J. Antimicrob. Chemother.*, 2003, 51, 605-612

[51] Chiang, T; Mariano, N; Urban, C; Colon-Urban, R; Grenner, L; Eng, RH; Huang, D; Dholakia, H; Rahal, JJ. Identification of carbapenem-resistant klebsiella pneumoniae harboring KPC enzymes in New Jersey. *Microb. Drug Resist.*, 2007, 13, 235-239.

[52] Hindiyeh, M; Smollen, G; Grossman, Z; Ram, D; Davidson, Y; Mileguir, F; Vax, M; Ben David, D; Tal, I; Rahav, G; Shamiss, A; Mendelson, E; Keller, N. Rapid detection of blaKPC carbapenamase genes by Real-Time PCR. *J. Clin. Microbiol.*, 2008 Jul 9. [Epub ahead of print]

[53] Deresinski, S. Vancomycin: does it still have a role as an antistaphylococcal agent? *Expert Rev. Anti Infect. Ther.*, 2007, 5, 393-401.

[54] Moellering RC, Jr; Krogstad, DJ; Greenblatt, DJ. Pharmacokinetics of vancomycin in normal subjects and in patients with reduced renal function. *Rev. Infect. Dis.*, 1981, 3 suppl, S230-235.

[55] Kasiakou, SK; Sermaides, GJ; Michalopoulos, A; Soteriades, ES; Falagas, ME. Continuous versus intermittent intravenous administration of antibiotics: a meta-analysis of randomised controlled trials. Lancet Infect Dis. 2005;5:581-589. acute micrococcal endocarditis. *Proc. Staff Meet Mayo Clin.*, 1958, 33, 172-181.

[56] Cantu, TG; Yamanaka-Yuen, NA; Lietman, PS. Serum vancomycin concentrations: reappraisal of their clinical value. *Clin. Infect Dis.,* 1994, 18, 533-543.

[57] Freeman, CD; Quintiliani, R; Nightingale, CH. Vancomycin therapeutic drug monitoring: is it necessary? *Ann. Pharmacother.*, 1993, 27, 594-598.

[58] Leader, WG; Chandler, MH; Castiglia, M. Pharmacokinetic optimisation of vancomycin therapy. *Clin. Pharmacokinet.*, 1995, 28, 327-342.

[59] Mellor, JA; Kingdom, J; Cafferkey, M; Keane, CT. Vancomycin toxicity: A prospective study. *J. Antimicrob. Chemother.*, 1985, 15, 773-780.

[60] Rybak, MJ; Albrecht, LM; Boike, SC; Chandrasekar, PH. Nephrotoxicity of vancomycin, alone and with an aminoglycoside. *J. Antimicrob. Chemotherapy.*, 1990, 25, 679-687.

[61] Downs, NJ; Neihart, RE; Dolezal, JM; Hodges, DR. Mild nephrotoxicity associated with vancomycin use. *Arch. Intern. Med.*, 1989, 149, 1777-1781.

[62] Wai, AO; Lo, AM; Abdo, A; Marra, F. Vancomycin-induced acute interstitial nephritis. *Ann. Pharmacother.*, 1998, 32, 1160-1164.

[63] Streetman, DS; Nafziger, AN; Destache, CJ; Bertino AS, Jr. Individualized pharmacokinetic monitoring results in less aminoglycoside-associated nephrotoxicity and fewer associated costs. *Pharmacotherapy.*, 2001, 21, 443-451.

[64] Karam, CM; McKinnon, PS; Neuhauser, MM; Rybak, MJ. Outcome assessment of minimizing vancomycin monitoring and dosing adjustments. *Pharmacotherapy.*, 1999, 19, 257-266.

[65] Darko, W; Medicis, JJ; Smith, A; Guharoy, R; Lehmann, DE. Mississippi mud no more: cost-effectiveness of pharmacokinetic dosage adjustment of vancomycin to prevent nephrotoxicity. *Pharmacotherapy.*, 2003, 5, 643-650.

[66] Malacarne, P; Bergamasco, S; Donadio, C. Nephrotoxicity due to combination antibiotic therapy with vancomycin and aminoglycosides in septic critically ill patients. *Chemotherapy.*, 2006, 52, 178-184.

[67] Hidayat, LK; Hsu, DI; Quist, R; Shriner, KA; Wong-Beringer, A. High-dose vancomycin therapy for methicillin-resistant Staphylococcus aureus infections: efficacy and toxicity. *Arch. Intern. Med.*, 2006, 166, 2138-2144.

[68] Vance-Bryan, K; Rotschafer, JC; Gilliland, SS; Rodvold, KA; Fitzgerald, CM; Guay, DR. A comparative assessment of vancomycin-associated nephrotoxicity in the young versus the elderly hospitalized patient. *J. Antimicrob. Chemother.*, 1994, 33, 811-821.

[69] Ingram, PR; Lye, DC; Tambyah, PA; Goh, WP; Tam, VH; Fisher, DA. Risk factors for nephrotoxicity associated with continuous vancomycin infusion in outpatient parenteral antibiotic therapy. *J. Antimicrob. Chemother.*, 2008, 62, 168-171.

[70] Lodise, TP; Lomaestro, B; Graves, J; Drusano, GL. Larger vancomycin doses (at least four grams per day) are associated with an increased incidence of nephrotoxicity. *Antimicrob. Agents Chemother.*, 2008, 52, 1330-1336.

[71] Geraci, JE. Vancomycin. *Mayo Clin. Proc.*, 1977, 52, 631-634.

[72] Wilhelm, MP; Estes, L. Vancomycin. *Mayo Clin. Proc.*, 1999, 74, 928-935.

[73] Iwamoto, T; Kagawa, Y; Kojima, M. Clinical efficacy of therapeutic drug monitoring in patients receiving vancomycin. *Biol. Pharm. Bull.*, 2003, 26, 876-879.

[74] Naschitz, JE; Gagarin, A; Gropper Schor, RE. Spurious Toxic Vancomycin Levels. *Eur. J. Intern. Med.*, 2008, 19, e36-37.

[75] Mackett, RL; Guay, DR. Vancomycin-induced neutropenia. *Can. Med. Assoc. J.*, 1985, 132, 39-40.

[76] Koo, KB; Bachand, RL; Chow, AW. Vancomycin-induced neutropenia. *Drug Intell. Clin. Pharm.*, 1986, 20, 780-782.

[77] Bernard, E; Perbost, I; Carles, M; Michiels, A; Carsenti-Etesse, H; Chichmanian, RM; Dunais, B; Dellamonica, P. Efficacy and safety of vancomycin constant-rate infusion in the treatment of chronic gram-positive bone and joint infections. *Clin. Microbiol. Infect.*, 1997, 3, 440-446.

[78] Pai, MP. Epidemiology of vancomycin-induced neutropenia in patients receiving home intravenous infusion therapy. *Ann. Pharmacother.*, 2006, 40, 224-228.

[79] Lai, KK; Kleinjan, J; Belliveau, P. Vancomycin-induced neutropenia treated with granulocyte colony-stimulating factor during home intravenous infusion therapy. *Clin. Infect. Dis.*, 1996, 23, 844-845.

[80] Bush, K; Heep, M; Macielag, MJ; Noel, GJ. Anti-MRSA beta-lactams in development, with a focus on ceftobiprole: the first anti-MRSA beta-lactam to demonstrate clinical efficacy. *Expert Opin. Investig. Drugs.*, 2007, 16, 419-429.

[81] Pan, A; Lorenzotti, S; Zoncada, A. Registered and investigational drugs for the treatment of methicillin-resistant Staphylococcus aureus infection. *Recent Patents Anti-Infect. Drug Disc.*, 2008, 3, 10-33.

[82] McDonald, LC. Trends in antimicrobial resistance in health care-associated pathogens and effect on treatment. *Clin. Infect. Dis.*, 2006, 42 Suppl 2, S65-71.

[83] Appelbaum, PC. MRSA--the tip of the iceberg. *Clin. Microbiol. Infect.*, 2006, 12, Suppl 2, 3-10.

[84] Sampathkumar, P. Methicillin-Resistant Staphylococcus aureus: The Latest Health Scare. *Mayo Clin. Proc.* 2007, 82, 1463-1414

[85] Tacconelli, E; Cataldo, MA. Vancomycin-resistant enterococci (VRE): transmission and control. *Int. J. Antimicrob. Agents.*, 2008, 31, 99-106.

[86] Siegel, JD; Rhinehart, E; Jackson, M; Chiarello, L; Health Care Infection Control Practices Advisory Committee. 2007 Guideline for Isolation Precautions: Preventing Transmission of Infectious Agents in Health Care Settings. *Am. J. Infect. Control.*, 2007, 35 (10 Suppl 2), S65-164.

[87] Safdar, N; Marx, J; Meyer, NA; Maki, DG. Effectiveness of preemptive barrier precautions in controlling nosocomial colonization and infection by methicillin-resistant Staphylococcus aureus in a burn unit. *Am. J. Infect. Control.*, 2006, 34, 476-483.

[88] West, TE; Guerry, C; Hiott, M; Morrow, N; Ward, K; Salgado, CD. Effect of targeted surveillance for control of methicillin-resistant Staphylococcus aureus in a community hospital system. *Infect. Control Hosp. Epidemiol.*, 2006, 27, 233-238.

[89] Eveillard, M; Eb, F; Tramier, B; Schmit, JL; Lescure, FX; Biendo, M; Canarelli, B; Daoudi, F; Laurans, G; Rousseau, F; Thomas, D. Evaluation of the contribution of isolation precautions in prevention and control of multi-resistant bacteria in a teaching hospital. *J. Hosp. Infect.*, 2001, 47, 116-124.

[90] Jaqua-Stewart, MJ; Tjaden, J; Humphreys, DW; Bade, P; Tille, PM; Peterson, KG; Salem, AG. Reduction in methicillin-resistant Staphylococcus aureus infection rate in a nursing home by aggressive containment strategies. *S. D. J. Med.,* 1999, 52, 241-247.

[91] Santos, RP; Mayo, TW; Siegel, JD. Healthcare epidemiology: active surveillance cultures and contact precautions for control of multidrug-resistant organisms: ethical considerations. *Clin. Infect. Dis.*, 2008, 47, 110-116.

[92] Aboelela, SW; Saiman, L; Stone, P; Lowy, FD; Quiros, D; Larson, E. Effectiveness of barrier precautions and surveillance cultures to control transmission of multidrug-resistant organisms: a systematic review of the literature. *Am. J. Infect. Control.*, 2006, 34, 484-494.

INDEX

C

D